ENDORSEMENTS

We don't get to choose all roads in life and can be confronted with uncertainty which we then need to navigate. Life can take an unexpected turn at any moment. What do you do when it is drastically interrupted? I found this book filled with hope and practical information. It inspires you to do your journey well, whatever that may be. Wendy's experiences and insights helps increase your faith to overcome adversities and challenges you or a loved one may face. This book is a valuable resource for any parent, spouse, caregiver, family or friend of a seriously ill child, teen or adult.

Lydia Quirey

Lydia is my friend who initially suggested I take Victoria to see a doctor. Five years later, her daughter was diagnosed with a life-threatening illness.

This book is a very helpful guide for parents who gather strength through their religion in times of severe challenge to assist them to maintain hope and sustain the energy needed to manage the treatment journey. It may also be helpful to those who might struggle with their faith during these times – particularly with relevant quotations from psalms...

... For those parents who prefer to find other ways to assist in staying strong, this book is full of lists of practical suggestions and plans which will save time and energy – both usually very scarce for most families. Wendy also lists the support resources available to all families support their children through brain cancer both through the text and in all appendices at the end of the book based on her own lived experience (including the mention of Redkite's telegroup program which is how I came to know her). Support strategies for siblings and for the child with cancer are there too.

"Victoria Grace" is also a very well written story of human strength and resilience – I couldn't put it down even though I knew the story. Thank you Wendy for providing so much meaningful assistance to other parents, extended family and support networks!

Linda Brown
Senior Social Worker – Redkite

Redkite is an Australian cancer charity providing essential support to children and young people (0-24 years) with cancer, and the family and support network who care for them.

*A free audio recording of the
Introduction and Chapter 1 can be downloaded from
Wendyrobinson.com.au*

Victoria Grace

Living with victory through childhood cancer

Wendy Robinson

VICTORIA GRACE

Copyright ©2018 by Wendy Robinson

All rights reserved. This book is protected by the copyright laws of Australia. This book may not be copied or reprinted for commercial gain or profit. The use of short quotations or occasional page copying for personal or group study is permitted and encouraged. Permission will be granted upon request, contact the author at wendy@wendyrobinson.com.au

The author and publisher are in no way liable for the misuse of any of the material.

All Scripture quotations, unless otherwise indicated, are taken from the Amplified® Bible (AMPC), Copyright © 1954, 1958, 1962, 1964, 1965, 1987 by The Lockman Foundation Used by permission.

Scripture quotations marked (ESV) are from The ESV® Bible (The Holy Bible, English Standard Version®), copyright © 2001 by Crossway, a publishing ministry of Good News Publishers. Used by permission. All rights reserved.

Scripture quotations marked (The Message) are taken from THE MESSAGE, copyright © 1993, 1994, 1995, 1996, 2000, 2001, 2002 by Eugene H. Peterson. Used by permission of NavPress. All rights reserved. Represented by Tyndale House Publishers, Inc.

Scripture quotations marked (NLT) are taken from the Holy Bible, New Living Translation, copyright ©1996, 2004, 2007, 2013, 2015 by Tyndale House Foundation. Used by permission of Tyndale House Publishers, Inc., Carol Stream, Illinois 60188. All rights reserved.

Scripture quotations marked (NKJV) are taken from the New King James Version®. Copyright © 1982 by Thomas Nelson. Used by permission. All rights reserved.

Scripture quotations marked (NIV) are taken from the Holy Bible, New International Version®, NIV®. Copyright © 1973, 1978, 1984, 2011 by Biblica, Inc.™ Used by permission of Zondervan. All rights reserved worldwide. www.zondervan.com The "NIV" and "New International Version" are trademarks registered in the United States Patent and Trademark Office by Biblica, Inc.™

Take note that the name satan and related names are not capitalised. We choose not to acknowledge him, even to the point of violating grammatical rules.

First published in Australia by Wendy Robinson, 2018

ISBN (978-0-6482476-0-9) Print Version

ISBN (978-0-6482476-1-6) eBook

ISBN (978-0-6482476-2-3) Audio Book

Cover design: Rebecca Heininger

Interior design: Rebecca Heininger

Front cover image: Victoria (4yrs), receiving her first chemotherapy treatment in July 2012

Back cover image: Victoria (5yrs), loving her Starlight Wish at Mt Buller, Victoria, in August 2013

Disclaimer

The author and publisher have made every effort to ensure the completeness and accuracy of information contained in this book; however, they assume no responsibilities for unwitting errors, omissions or inaccuracies.

This book is intended for educational purposes only. It is not intended as a substitue for diagnosis, treatment, or advice from your qualified practitioner. The facts presented in the following pages are offered as information only, not medical advice. If you have cancer, or if you are concerned about cancer, you should seek professional advice. If you have hemiplegia, you should seek professional advice. If you have depression or if you are concerned about depression, you should seek professional advice.

The author assumes no responsibility for inaccuracies in the source materials, nor in how this material is used. This is not intended to be a comprehensive book, thus it does not claim to contain information on all the possible therapies that could be used for or in relation to cancer, hemiplegia or mental illness.

*This book is dedicated to our daughter,
Victoria Grace, without whom
there would have been no story to write.*

I love you Victoria.

*Thank you for showing me how to
live in victory despite my circumstances.*

TABLE OF CONTENTS

Introduction 13

Chapter 1 – The Diagnosis 17
    Christmas Holidays 17
    Reflection - The importance of a shared faith
    when the going gets tough 33

Chapter 2 – Family, Fun and Fear 41
    Waiting Days 41
    Reflection - Distractions - there is a battle going on 66

Chapter 3 – Post Op Recovery 71
    Hospital and waiting days 71
    Reflection - The Holy Spirit – our Comforter 86

Chapter 4 – Home and Rehabilitation 93
    Emails from 8th Feb to 3rd Mar 2011 93
    Reflection – Rehab – Conquering and creativity 105

Chapter 5 – More Therapy 115
    Emails from 14th Mar to 18th May 2011 115
    Reflection – Creativity in therapy 127

Chapter 6 – New Things and Events 133
    Emails from 16th Jun 2011 to 30th Jan 2012 133
    Reflection – Camp Quality meets our needs 142

Chapter 7 – The News We Didn't Want 147

Emails from 22nd Feb to 18th Jun 2012 147
Reflection – Dealing with disappointment 159

Chapter 8 – Chemotherapy 163
Emails from 19th Jun to 22nd Jul 2012 163
Reflection – The Carer needs to be cared for 171

Chapter 9 – Wonderful Support 181
Emails from 1st Aug to 14th Sep 2012 181
Reflection – Community, giving and receiving 193

Chapter 10 – Scans and A Big Scare 199
Emails from 1st Oct to 16th Nov 2012 199
Reflection – Plan B preparing for the crisis 207

Chapter 11 – The Silly Season 215
Emails from 26th Nov to 28th Dec 2012 215
Reflection – Mothers 227

Chapter 12 – New Year and a Blog 233
Emails from 6th Jan to 24th Jan 2013 233
Reflection – Writing as therapy 244

Chapter 13 – School and Another MRI 249
Blog posts – 31st Jan to 15th Feb 2013 249
Reflection – Fathers 263

Chapter 14 – Normal Life 269
Blog posts – 19th Feb to 29th Mar 2013 269
Reflection – Siblings are a blessing 286

Chapter 15 – Living From Scan to Scan 295
    Blog posts – 9th Apr to 21st May 2013 295
    Reflection – Thankfulness is key 311

Chapter 16 – High Temperatures and Hospital Again 317
    Blog posts – 29th May to 5th Jul 2013 317
    Reflection – Practical tips for the home of a
    child on chemo 333

Chapter 17 – Precious Family Time 341
    Blog posts – 12th Jul to 26th Jul 2013 341
    Reflection – The Bible 356

Chapter 18 – The Wish 361
    Blog posts – 3rd Aug to 9th Aug 2013 361
    Reflection – Charities 369

Chapter 19 – Reality Hits Fast 375
    Blog posts – 11th Aug to 19th Sep 2013 375
    Reflection – Keeping the left leg working 392

Chapter 20 – Living From a Place of Victory 399
    Blog posts – 27th Sep to 29th Oct 2013 399
    Final Reflection – Three years of learning 411

Epilogue 419

Acknowledgements 421

About Wendy Robinson 425

Appendix A: Scriptures.. *427*

Appendix B: Victoria's Medical Diagnoses............................. *433*

Appendix C: Occupational Therapy Activities *437*

Appendix D: One Hour Occupational Therapy Plan *445*

Appendix E: Master List of Lists *447*

Appendix F: Emergency Hospital Bag Contents Checklist..... *449*

Appendix G: Homecoming Checklist *451*

Appendix H: School Booklet.. *453*

Appendix I: Signs for Displaying at Home *465*

Appendix J: Home Medical Kit *469*

Appendix K: Charities that have helped our family................ *471*

Appendix L: Maintaining and Improving Leg Function *473*

Notes *477*

*Yet amid all these things
we are more than conquerors
and gain a surpassing victory
through Him Who loved us.*

(Romans 8:37)

INTRODUCTION

What's going to happen to our daughter? How do I tell my husband?

I desperately wanted the doctor's words to be wrong. I wanted to do a delete of the last six hours and return to our normal, slightly chaotic life as a family of six. But we don't live in a fantasy world. This was reality. I had just been told that our three year old child had a mass in her brain.

I want this all to go away. I can't believe this is happening to us. I'm frightened.

Perhaps you've had thoughts similar to these during a tough time in your life. Or you could be thinking them right now.

Fear, pain, anger and grief may be consuming you. I have felt these emotions many times during our journey of having a child with a brain tumour and its ongoing implications.

Fear of what could happen to our child and how we as a family would make it through; the pain of witnessing a child who was seemingly healthy suddenly become physically disabled, requiring hours of rehabilitation; Anger, asking why did this happen to our child? And the grief of witnessing a childhood that was no longer carefree.

But alongside these emotions there has also been perseverance, faith, hope and love. Perseverance to do all that was possible to help our child physically and emotionally; A rising faith, although wavering at times, faith to believe that there is a God in Heaven who is on our side; Increasing hope in a God who has a plan that is good; Learning to receive love, the love of family, friends, church family, school community, neighbours and the love of strangers through charities. But most importantly the love of Jesus Christ, who laid down His life for us so we could confidently declare Romans 8:37, Yet in all these things we are more than conquerors through Him who loved us (NKJV).

This book chronologically covers the first three years of our journey of having a child with a brain tumour. During that time, I as the mother, have learned much including strategies to help care for the emotional and physical needs of a child on chemotherapy, and who also has hemiplegia (left side weakness); as well as strategies to overcome the mental health strain of being a primary carer; and to maintain a marriage and care for the emotional well-being of our other three children. None of this we have done perfectly, but we have by the grace of God, made it through to the other side with our family still together!

At the end of each chapter there is a reflection in which I have endeavoured to explain these strategies along with examples of how we implemented them. In the

INTRODUCTION

appendices I have included the practical checklists I created for our family and those who lovingly came to help in our home. These checklists enabled us to keep some sense of order in the chaos. If you've found yourself on a similar journey to us, my prayer is that the inclusion of these practical strategies and checklists will be of great benefit to you and your family.

Finally, as you read our story, I pray that you will be encouraged to persevere despite the fear, pain, anger and grief. And that you will be inspired to grow in faith and hope, and fully receive the love offered to you by other people and Jesus Christ.

Chapter 1

The Diagnosis

CHRISTMAS HOLIDAYS

Christmas day had arrived at last. Charlotte and Victoria couldn't wait to do their concert for the family. Aged five and three, they just loved to entertain. We even made posters and displayed them around our home to advertise 'The Charlotte and Victoria Show.' Marshall, who at seven years old was more interested in playing with his Lego, reluctantly sat down to watch the show. Alexandra, thirteen months old, was having her afternoon sleep and was oblivious to all the commotion. My husband Ken and I sat down anticipating what our stage-bound daughters would amuse us with this afternoon.

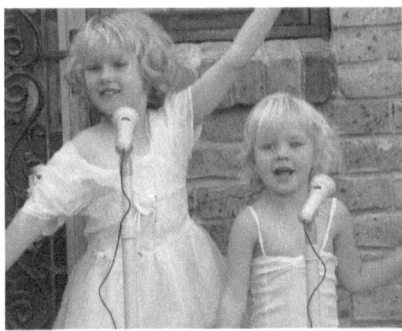

Charlotte and Victoria at home performing their Christmas Day concert. Oh how I would look back at this photo and see what I hadn't seen at the time.

A week later, after the New Year's Eve celebrations to welcome in 2011, we headed off to Lemon Tree Passage at Port Stephens, NSW. Wonderful family memories were created. The children spent hours riding around on their bikes.

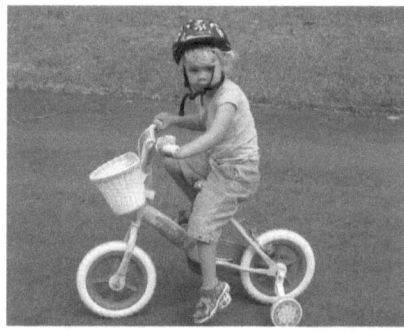

Victoria riding her bike at Lemon Tree Passage Again I would look at this photo and wonder, why didn't we notice Victoria was unable to hold her left wrist up?

After returning from Lemon Tree Passage, we headed down to the Sydney Aquarium to see the Lego exhibition.

While we were walking around, Victoria kept saying, 'I can't walk properly.' She was constantly falling over. After telling her numerous times, 'Just slow down and watch where you are going,' I stopped and studied how she was walking.

What I saw was a bit concerning. Victoria had virtually no control over her left foot. When she took a step with her left leg, her foot turned completely inwards. Her left foot was at right angles to her right foot. Victoria had no strength to point her left foot forward. Well, how bad did I feel with my, 'Just slow down and watch where you are going,' comment? Clearly there was something amiss with her foot or leg or hip. Or so we thought.

On the way home from Sydney, Ken and I discussed a course of action. Being a Saturday night, our local doctor's surgery was closed, so we decided that as soon as we got home, Ken would take Victoria to a nearby after hours medical centre. They returned from the medical centre with instructions to come back on Sunday morning to get a hip x-ray done.

On Tuesday, I took Victoria to the medical centre to get the X-Ray results. The doctor advised that all looked fine in the X-Ray, however, as the walking problem was still evident, he advised me to get an ultrasound of Victoria's left hip. We were able to get the ultrasound done onsite immediately at the medical centre. Her hip looked normal. The doctor advised that we return in a couple of weeks so he could review her walking. That sounded like a reasonable course of action to me at the time.

WEDNESDAY 19TH JANUARY 2011

The very next afternoon we met up with some friends at the beach. It was a glorious day. As we were walking to the park at the beach, my very observant friend, who is a nurse, asked me, 'What's going on with Victoria's walking?'

I nonchalantly replied, 'Oh, we have been to the doctor

and he thinks it is some kind of hip problem, so we are just waiting to see what happens over the next few weeks.'

My gracious friend said to me, 'I think there is something else happening. Can you see how her left shoulder is drooping too?'

'Oh yes,' I replied, still blissfully unaware of what that critical observation meant.

We chatted for about half an hour about other events going on in our lives. Then my friend tactfully said to me, 'I think you should take Victoria to your GP (General Practitioner) in the morning to get her looked at again.'

'Okay,' I replied, 'If you think so.'

Then my beautiful friend offered to come over and look after the other children while I took Victoria to the doctor. At this point I was starting to feel a little uneasy. I wondered why my friend was offering to help to look after the other children. Couldn't they just come with me like they normally do? I phoned my GP and made an appointment for the next morning. So with a plan in place, the children played in the surf for another hour or so before we packed up and left for home.

On the 30 minute drive home, my friend's carefully chosen words went continually round and round in my head. The look of concern on her face, even though she had tried to

THE DIAGNOSIS

hide it, filled my mind. Why was she so concerned about Victoria? Why did she want to come over and look after the children while I took Victoria to our GP?

By the time I was 5 minutes away from home, I had worked myself into quite a distressed state. I decided not to wait until the morning to find out what was wrong with Victoria, but rather thought I would seek advice from a friend's husband who was a doctor. I knew he would know what we needed to do. So I drove straight past our house, parked in their driveway and ran up to the front door. With tears rolling down my face, I said, 'There is something wrong with Victoria.'

Once again the grace shown to me was unforgettable. My friend's husband did a few observations of Victoria and then spoke briefly to his wife. He told me to take Victoria to the John Hunter Hospital straightaway, and when I got there, I was to tell the emergency department staff that he had checked Victoria out and said she needed to be seen immediately. Ken was on his way to Melbourne for a business trip, so my friend kindly offered to look after our other three children at home.

By this time, I was desperately concerned about Victoria. I was still unsure as to what was going on with her, but was getting a strong impression from my friends that it was something very serious. We left the medical centre only one day ago with, 'Just come back in four to six weeks', and now I was being told, 'Victoria needs to go to the hospital straightaway.' My mind was racing, while I was trying to stay calm for Victoria's sake.

I had never been to the John Hunter Hospital before. I didn't even know where to park, let alone know where the Emergency Department was. I finally managed to find a park, in the car park furthest away from the Emergency Department. Victoria had to walk as best as she could along a seemingly endless corridor.

When we eventually found the Emergency Department, I explained to the triage nurse what had happened and mentioned our doctor friend's name. The staff swung into action rather quickly and we were whisked into the Emergency rooms.

By this time it was 7pm. Thankfully Victoria had asked to bring a balloon from the car into the hospital. The balloon provided hours of entertainment, actually four hours, as she was assessed by numerous doctors. Lots of strength tests were performed, including Victoria wrapping her fingers around the doctor's finger and squeezing tight; and pushing with the sole of feet against doctor's hands. There was plenty of testing Victoria's arms and legs with the reflex hammer too.

At around 11pm, a neurologist came to see us. It was her first day at John Hunter Hospital. 'We are arranging for Victoria to have a CT (Computed Tomography) scan tonight,' she said.

THE DIAGNOSIS

I was beginning to understand that this was a much bigger problem than Victoria being unable to walk properly.

Preparation for the CT scan included the insertion of a cannula into her hand, a traumatic experience for both her and me. Finally at midnight, we walked into the room with the CT scanner. Victoria was still awake, chatting to everyone.

As she lay on the bed to go into the machine, I stood beside her with a protective vest on. I prayed, 'God please give her and us the strength to get through this, whatever the outcome.'

As I now reflect on this moment, there was some similarity to when in the book of Genesis in the Bible, Abraham put Isaac on the altar.

> *'Don't lay a hand on that boy! Don't touch him! Now I know how fearlessly you fear God; you didn't hesitate to place your son, your dear son, on the altar for me.' Abraham looked up. He saw a ram caught by its horns in the thicket. Abraham took the ram and sacrificed it as a burnt offering instead of his son. Abraham named that place GOD-Yireh (GOD-Sees-To-It). That's where we get the saying, 'On the mountain of GOD, he sees to it.'*
> (Genesis 22:12-14 The Message)

Of course there was at least one big difference: Abraham

laid Isaac on the altar in obedience to God. I had laid Victoria out on the bed of the CT scanner, which may as well have been an altar, at the request of the neurologist. However, we were both in a position of having to trust God completely with the life of our children. We had to trust that God would see to it.

When the CT scan was finished the neurologist walked us back to a room in the Emergency Department. Not a curtained bay like the one we were originally in, but a proper room with a door that could be shut. During the scan Victoria had finally fallen asleep and was blissfully unaware of the words that were about to be spoken. I sat looking at my child, thinking, 'Thankfully she has gone to sleep. She will be so tired tomorrow.'

The neurologist came into the room and simply said, 'The CT scan showed that there is a mass in your child's brain.'

'No!' I screamed, and started to sob.

The neurologist explained the next steps to me, which included an MRI (Magnetic Resonance Imaging) in the morning. Frankly I cannot remember much else of what she said. All I was thinking was, how can this be? This child is so well and healthy. Why didn't we notice before? Was there something we could have done to detect this earlier?

However, I do remember these words from the Neurologist, and am very grateful for them. 'If you had brought her

THE DIAGNOSIS

here earlier, last week or last month, it would have made no difference.' By saying that she immediately removed any feelings of guilt regarding us not reacting quickly enough to the symptoms Victoria had been displaying.

I couldn't contemplate phoning Ken in Melbourne with this news. I asked the Neurologist to call and explain it all to him, as I sat there in complete shock. Ken was aware we were at the hospital as on the way here I had phoned both him and my mother, to let them know that we were going to get Victoria's leg problem sorted out. But now we were facing a completely different scenario.

After ten minutes or so, I managed to summon the strength to phone my Mum in New Zealand. All I could say to her was, 'Mum, I need you here now.'

Being the wonderful mother she is, she was on the first plane out of New Zealand the next morning.

Victoria was moved from the Emergency Department and taken down to the J1 Children's Oncology Ward to spend the night there, our first night of many. She didn't get much sleep due to the required four hourly observations. As for my night's sleep, I really can't remember if I got any sleep or not. Perhaps I had a couple of hours from sheer emotional exhaustion.

> *For anyone who is wondering if we took any action regarding the initial misdiagnosis of Victoria's illness, in February 2011 we lodged a complaint with the Health Care Complaints Commission. The main outcome we wanted was for the doctor to be aware of his misdiagnosis, with the view to preventing future misdiagnoses of brain tumours when physical symptoms are present. From subsequent correspondence with the Health Care Complaints Commission, it appears that this outcome was achieved.*

THURSDAY 20TH JANUARY 2011

On Thursday morning the doctors were milling around the Nurses' Station outside Victoria's room, studying her CT scans. I say 'doctors,' as there were about eight of them. They were chatting among themselves about what would be the best course of action. I was a bit taken aback by such an 'open air' discussion. Having worked in the corporate sphere prior to having children, I was used to meetings of any significance being held behind closed doors. Clearly that was not the approach taken here. The Nurses' Station in the middle of the ward was the place where it all happened.

THE DIAGNOSIS

I stood by, trying to glean what information I could. One doctor's comment sticks in my mind.

It was something like, 'We should do an MRI of her spine as well as her brain, just in case there is anything there too.'

Hearing that was too much for me. I retreated back to Victoria's room and continued distracting her from the frustration of not being able to eat or drink. The MRI of the brain and spine required Victoria to lie completely still for about 40 minutes. This was a big ask for a three year old. So the doctors arranged for Victoria to have a general anaesthetic just prior to the MRI. This meant that she was assigned 'nil by mouth' status until the scan had been completed. Victoria had not eaten or drunk anything since about 5pm the previous day.

Finally at around 2pm she had the MRI. Needless to say, it was a very long and tedious day, filled with hours of placating and finding creative distractions.

My mum arrived just after the scan was completed. How wonderful it was to have Mum there so she could take over the care of Victoria while I sat with the doctors. There was another meeting at the Nurses' Station. This time I wasn't on the fringes, but sitting right in the middle of the meeting, being given all the details of what was happening in Victoria's brain. There was no retreating now.

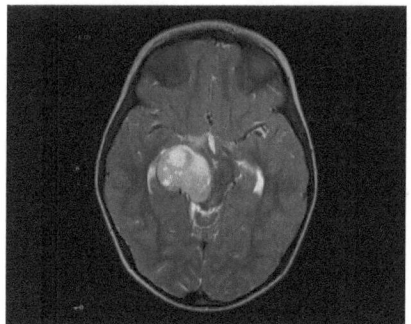

MRI of the tumour in Victoria's brain on 20th January 2011

One of the doctors said to me, 'This is a very unusual tumour, in a very unusual place.'

Those weren't exactly the words I wanted to hear. It appeared the tumour was 3 to 4 cm in size, sort of like a golf ball. It was low to the right of centre in Victoria's brain, positioned on, or attached to, her brain stem.

The tumour was pressing on the right side of her brain. The pressure was causing left sided weakness, meaning reduced strength in her leg, foot, arm and hand on the left side; hence the reason she had been having so much difficulty walking.

One of the biggest concerns the doctors had was how to access the tumour while doing minimal damage to Victoria's brain. The surgeon was going to canvas opinions on the best surgical approach from experts around the world.

My sister, her husband and child arrived at the hospital

THE DIAGNOSIS

during this meeting. I will never forget the relief I felt when I saw my sister walk into the ward, pushing her child's stroller down the corridor. We needed all the support possible. Our world was turning upside down.

After hearing all the doctors had to say, I asked a close friend to pray with me. We went to the Quiet Room in the Ronald McDonald Family Room. What a blessing that room was to us during those two weeks in hospital. A lot of prayers were said there.

As soon as we sat down in the Quiet Room, I put my head in my hands and sobbed and sobbed.

I literally cried out to God, 'Please God we need a miracle, I know this little girl is your daughter, and she is 'on loan' to us. Please give these doctors wisdom.'

During that time of being utterly distraught, this psalm came to mind,

> 'May we shout for joy over your victory and lift up our banners in the name of our God. May the LORD grant all your requests.'
> (Psalm 20:5 NIV)

Around 8pm that night, Ken arrived back from Melbourne. He came straight from Newcastle airport to the hospital. We hugged, cried and prayed.

FRIDAY 21ST JANUARY 2011

It was decided that Victoria would have brain surgery the following week. Brain surgery is certainly not minor surgery. One doctor told us that the best scenario from the operation was that the tumour would just pop out cleanly, leaving no damage to Victoria's brain. The worst scenario would be that as they cut into the tumour, it would bleed out and Victoria would die. Or the outcome could be something in the middle of these two scenarios. We had no choice but to wait and pray.

Later that morning, we met with a social worker, well actually the Head of the Social Work Department, as the paediatric social worker was on leave. He was the perfect person to help us. He spoke to us about many things, including gently telling us that this would be a long journey and that at every step along the journey we would have new things to deal with. He also said that we didn't both have to be in the hospital 24 hours, seven days a week, unless something critical was happening. This was very 'releasing' for both of us to hear. He spoke about the importance of having other adult support both at home and at the hospital, especially until we knew what the treatment plan was going to be. Thankfully we had that one covered with the amazing support of family, friends, neighbours, church and school.

We also discussed the practicalities of having a seriously ill child, the impact on family finances, and support services

THE DIAGNOSIS

available to help with electricity bills, telephone bills, car registration etc. One of the most practical pieces of advice he gave us was to be at the hospital by 9am so we could get a car park.

He gave us some insight into some of the behaviours we could expect from our other children, such as separation anxiety and an increased dependence upon Ken and me. His advice to us was to let them talk, trust in their ability to adapt and keep it simple. He reminded us that it was important we take time out as a couple and keep trying to do normal family things.

The social worker also spoke to us about our possible reactions to our situation. He helped us to understand that we would each react differently, and that was okay. The important thing was that we respect each other's reactions. It was another very wise piece of advice, as I am an internal processor, while Ken is an external processor. I wanted to hide in a room and share my thoughts and fears with God alone. Ken wanted to get on the phone and share the updates and his fears with family and friends. Both approaches were valid. We needed to acknowledge our differences, be gracious with each other, and give each other the freedom to manage our emotions our own way.

After this meeting, I had a whole new appreciation for social workers. Having never come into contact with them before, I got a glimpse of how very valuable their role was, giving support and advice in times of crisis. The social worker also met with some of our extended family, which not only acknowledged their important role as carers of us, but also offered them much needed support.

At Friday lunch time, as Victoria was healthy in every other way, the doctors told us we could take her home for the next five days. How grateful we were to hear those words. We couldn't get out of the hospital fast enough, so we could be in our own familiar environment and regroup as a family. The doctors said we had to return to the hospital immediately if Victoria started having headaches or vomiting.

What a blessing it was to walk out of the hospital that afternoon. We knew there was a very challenging road ahead. But we also knew that we now had potentially five days in which we could be a 'normal' family. We did not know what our future would hold past next Thursday, the day of Victoria's brain surgery.

As we drove home from the hospital, with the social worker's comments in mind about 'doing normal family things', Ken and I discussed what we would like to do in those five days to create the best family memories possible. We agreed on these three activities. Firstly, for Charlotte and Victoria to give us a re-run of their Christmas day concert. Secondly, go to church as a family and have the Elders pray for Victoria. Thirdly, go to the beach with our extended family, most of who were now either with us or on their way to visit.

REFLECTION - THE IMPORTANCE OF A SHARED FAITH WHEN THE GOING GETS TOUGH

Ken and I had been married for about twelve and a half years when Victoria was diagnosed. Prior to our marriage Ken had shared his Christian faith very openly with me. He was very blunt on a couple of occasions, saying,

'Your life is a mess. You need God.'

I found this quite offensive and for a while I would literally run the other way when I saw him.

I did have some knowledge of God. When I was a child growing up in New Zealand, my mother had taken me to church and I had started to develop a relationship with God. However, Marxist feminist teaching at university strongly influenced me, and in my late teens I stopped praying and stopped going to church.

So when Ken started talking to me about God, I simply said, 'I am not interested,' and changed the conversation.

I had my own thoughts on life. I was one of those Kiwis who, in my early twenties, moved to Sydney looking for work. After four years of working extremely hard and enjoying life in Sydney's Eastern Suburbs, I achieved my goal of buying an art deco apartment in Sydney's Elizabeth Bay. I couldn't wait to move in and feel the satisfaction of attaining my goal.

Well what a shock I got. As I lay in bed in my apartment on the first night, I realised I didn't feel any different to the night before when I was in the rental accommodation. The disappointment I felt was immense. A voice inside my head kept asking, 'Why do I feel so empty after all my hard work?'

Around that same time I attended a corporate retreat where we were asked to assess each area of our life. I was able to score ten out of ten for every area in my life, except Spirituality. To be completely honest, I had to put a zero in that box.

Being a task focussed person, I thought I had better fix this. However, little did I know that God was already on the case. The lady that gave me my first job in Sydney was a Christian. She had been praying for me diligently every day for three years.

As I searched for something to fill that spiritual void, I kept hearing that voice in my head saying. 'What is your life about Wendy? Buying the apartment didn't bring the satisfaction you were looking for. What is your vision? What is your purpose in life?' I couldn't answer these questions. I was gradually coming to the realisation that I didn't feel satisfied with my life. It felt empty. I had no vision and no purpose.

One day while walking to work, I eventually yielded to that still small voice. I called out to Jesus, 'OK, I give up doing life my way. I'll do it Your way.'

THE DIAGNOSIS

Immediately I felt the peace that I had thought buying the apartment would bring me. It was a true moment of revelation. I knew I was now on the right path, the path to a purposeful life. Later that day, I phoned Ken and asked if I could go to church with him. Three weeks later we were dating. Eighteen months later we were married.

At our wedding in June 1998 a friend, Neale Joseph, gave us one of his beautiful paintings, entitled 'Come to the Garden'. On the back of the painting he had made reference to some scriptures including one from Ecclesiastes:

> *Two are better than one, because they have a good [more satisfying] reward for their labour; For if they fall, the one will lift up his fellow. But woe to him who is alone when he falls and has not another to lift him up! Again, if two lie down together, then they have warmth; but how can one be warm alone? And though a man might prevail against him who is alone, two will withstand him. A threefold cord is not quickly broken.*
> (Ecclesiastes 4:9-12)

How true this scripture has been for our marriage. There have been many times since Victoria was diagnosed when Ken and I did not know what was going to happen next. There was nothing practical that we could do to change or improve Victoria's circumstance. We each responded very differently to the crisis. But there was one effective thing we could always do, and we could do it together – pray.

As marriage counsellors Dennis & Barbara Rainey said,

> *… God intends for marriage to be a spiritual relationship consisting of three – not just a man and a woman, but the two of them and their God relating spiritually and remaining committed to each other for a lifetime. Wouldn't it be natural for God, the One who initiated the relationship, to want a couple to bring their troubles, worries, and praises to Him on a regular, daily basis?'* [1]

I wonder how our responses would have differed if we hadn't shared the same faith? For a start, we wouldn't have been able to pray together. I can picture the conversation, or conflict, now …

'Why are you bothering to pray? What difference will that make? There isn't anybody listening.'

Praise God we had already worked through that basic truth fourteen years before, and God had brought us together in complete unity. We wouldn't have been able to genuinely quote scripture to each other as we prayed. Philippians 4:6-7 was a favourite.

> *Do not fret or have any anxiety about anything, but in every circumstance and in everything, by*

prayer and petition (definite requests), with thanksgiving, continue to make your wants known to God. And God's peace [shall be yours, that tranquil state of a soul assured of its salvation through Christ, and so fearing nothing from God and being content with its earthly lot of whatever sort that is, that peace] which transcends all understanding shall garrison and mount guard over your hearts and minds in Christ Jesus. (Philippians 4:6-7)

If we hadn't been looking to the same Source for the answers, it would have been challenging to trust that the decisions we were making were the right ones. We would have been relying on our own incomplete and differing knowledge, rather than submitting to God and his will.

We wouldn't have shared and encouraged each other with that deep knowing that God was with us in this situation, regardless of how devastating it seemed.

We can look back now and see that God had been preparing us for this time. Prior to Victoria's diagnosis our marriage had been good, but nowhere near perfect. We had gone through two miscarriages after Marshall's birth, and had to learn how to deal with grief and disappointment. We had to come to a place where we had the faith to believe that God would give us more children. And He did, three more, born almost two years and two weeks apart: Charlotte in September 2005,

Victoria in October 2007 and then Alexandra in November 2009, making our family complete. Financially we had experienced times of struggle as we navigated through the tribulations of owning a small business.

Both these times, and many others, had taught us the value of prayer, as well as the importance of coming together in unity, with thanksgiving, and submitting our requests to God. Especially in the times when we could do or say nothing other than,

'Please help us God, we don't know what to do.'

God would always answer, most often not as we expected. For fourteen years we had been learning how to wait for God's perfect timing, although we didn't always wait patiently and peacefully. But we waited. Stormie Omartian talks about this in her book, The Power of a Praying Wife, one of the first books I read when we got married. While Stormie is specifically talking about husbands and marriage, I believe these principals apply to all our prayers.

> *Above all, don't give place to impatience. Seeing answers to your prayers can take time, especially if your marriage is deeply wounded or strained. Be patient to persevere and wait for God to heal. Keep in mind that you are both imperfect people. Only the Lord is perfect. Look to God as the source of all you want to see happen in your marriage,*

> *and don't worry about how it will happen. It's your responsibility to pray. It's God's job to answer. Leave it in His hands.* [2]

I am grateful to God that He used Ken, and other precious people, to bring me to a place of repentance and acknowledgement of the need for Jesus in my life. I am grateful that He chose Ken to be my husband as God knew, all those years ago when we married, what was to come. He knew that our faith and trust in Him needed to be strengthened, so that when this challenge came into our lives, we would go to only one place – Him, and that we would go together.

> *I also tell you this: If two of you agree here on earth concerning anything you ask, my Father in heaven will do it for you. For where two or three gather together as my followers, I am there among them.* (Matthew 18:19-20 NLT)

Chapter 2

Family, Fun and Fear

WAITING DAYS

SATURDAY 22ND JANUARY 2011

How wonderful it was to wake up at home on Saturday morning, rather than in the hospital. We were confident that the surgeon would do his very best for our daughter, and even more confident that our God would get us all through, no matter what the outcome. However, in the midst of this trauma, I was still a mum with very raw emotions. It was my daughter who was in a fight for her life.

It was a beautiful summer morning and I went for a ride on my bike. As soon as I rode down the driveway, the tears began to flood. I called out to God, with an ache in my heart, 'She is only three years old, why does she have to go through this?'

I spent the next thirty minutes riding around our local streets, pouring out my heart to God. I returned home with peace in my heart and the strength from God to continue through the day.

The rest of the family was still sleeping when I returned from my ride. So I sat down with my journal and began thanking God for all the good things about this horrendous circumstance. I came up with a list of twenty two things to thank God for.

My list included things like friends with the specific knowledge needed for the diagnosis after the initial doctor's misdiagnosis. My mum's renewed passport arriving on the day of diagnosis, so she was able to be with us on the following day. Victoria's health and well-being, aside from the impact of the tumour, she was healthy and not in any pain. My sister and her family, who lived in New Zealand at the time, just happened to be holidaying in Byron Bay, Australia. They had planned to visit us the following week, so they came down a week earlier. Marshall's school teacher had already been in contact with parents via email, two weeks before the first term of 2011 commenced, which meant I was able to email her about our situation, and she called on the Junior School teachers to pray. I had finished breastfeeding Alexandra in December, so didn't have to do a quick painful wean. Earlier in the week I had done a lot of cooking for school lunches. The freezer was full of muffins and cupcakes.

To help keep us focussed on God and not our circumstance, I made some signs saying, 'This is a big trust God time,' and laminated them. I placed them all around our home. One was outside our front door, so anyone coming into our home would know Who we were putting our trust in at this very distressing time. I positioned another one in our back courtyard next to the back door, so while we were sitting outside having meals we could again be reminded to keep our focus on God, not our circumstances. And I put one on the wall next to our bed, so when I went to sleep at night I would remember that Victoria was His daughter too and God loved her more than we did.

By Saturday afternoon, our extended family, including my Dad who had come from New Zealand that day, were all at our home. We enjoyed an afternoon of fun in the pool, followed by the re-run of the Charlotte and Victoria Christmas concert, although there was slightly different choreography. Victoria relished every moment of it, especially being surrounded by all her family. Everyone appreciated the significance of this time together, doing their best to act like everything was normal, knowing very well that it was anything but normal.

Later that evening, Ken and I managed to sneak away for an hour to sit by the lake. We talked and prayed about next Thursday. We felt remarkably calm considering what we were about to face. We knew in our hearts that we could trust our God to get us through this circumstance, even if the outcome wasn't what we wanted.

Throughout this time, we continued to pray and declare Victoria Grace's name over her life. Victoria, meaning victor and conqueror and Grace, meaning blessing and favour. Before she was born, God had given me this name for her. He knew what would be needed to be declared every time we spoke her name. How imperative that was right now.

SUNDAY 23RD JANUARY 2011

With one of the activities for the weekend ticked off the list, we moved on to the next one, taking Victoria to church for a special time of prayer. As Christians, we believe what The Bible says in The Letter of James:

> *Is anyone among you sick? Let them call the elders of the church to pray over them and anoint them with oil in the name of the Lord.* (James 5:14 NIV)

On Sunday morning we went to church as normal, except it wasn't a normal morning. Ken had spoken with our pastor, who wisely suggested that we arrive late to church, avoiding any unwanted conversations or attention, and that we leave early from the service for the same reason. We were very grateful for his wisdom in this situation. It was hard enough having conversations among our family, let alone with other people. It was great having our entire extended family join us at church that morning for extra support.

During the service, Victoria was prayed over and anointed

with oil. It was another profoundly emotional moment for us all, as we acknowledged God's sovereignty over her life and asked for His healing power to pervade her body. We left the church service filled with faith and assurance that God was in the midst and He would prevail.

Sunday afternoon was the perfect time to action number three on the list, a visit to the beach. So after lunch, we all went to the beach - grandparents, aunts, uncle and cousins. The adults understood the significance of the family outing, valiantly keeping smiles on our faces, trying not to focus on what lay ahead. I remember watching Victoria jumping over the little waves as best she could and all I could think was, 'Will she be able to still do this after the operation?'

The weekend had seemingly been a perfect family time together. Except, of course, for the reason we were all there. We had created the types of memories you would expect from a Christmas holiday, not a lead up to brain surgery. The three family activities Ken and I had wanted to do were done. Just as well, as the supposed seven days at home was about to be cut short.

MONDAY 24TH JANUARY 2011

At One o'clock Monday morning, Victoria woke up crying and complaining about a headache. We phoned the hospital and they said to bring her in immediately, so I hurriedly packed our bags. Victoria, Ken and I returned to the J1 ward at the John Hunter Hospital. Thankfully we had extended family staying in our home so they were able to take care of Marshall, Charlotte and Alexandra. No doubt it would have been quite disconcerting for them to wake in the morning to find Mum, Dad and Victoria gone. It added further confusion and uncertainty to their already troubled minds.

By morning, the headaches had subsided. After doing his rounds, the doctor gave us a choice. We could go home, and return to hospital if the headaches came back. Or we could stay in the hospital until the operation, which was scheduled for early Thursday morning. We were fearful that if we went home we might miss a vital symptom indicating things were worsening for Victoria, jeopardising her well-being further. Hospital was where we decided to stay, surrounded by professionals who knew what symptoms to watch for. We felt safer in the hospital environment.

Staying in hospital also meant less upheaval for our other three children. If we went home and then had to return to hospital again in the middle of the night, their stress would only increase. With Victoria, Ken and me in hospital, the other children could continue with some of the school holiday activities we had planned. Their life could remain as normal as possible, albeit interwoven with visits to see their sister in hospital.

For the next three days, both Ken and I stayed at the

hospital with Victoria. We wanted to ensure she felt as safe and peaceful as possible about the upcoming surgery. Even though she was only three, she was obviously aware that something was wrong with her body, as she couldn't walk properly and she couldn't use her left hand. I slept in the room with Victoria. Ken slept in the vacant palliative care room down the hallway.

I remember finding it very difficult to walk into the ward, seeing the word 'Oncology' on the wall. I thought, 'How did we get here?'

Two weeks ago we were having the ideal family holiday at Lemon Tree Passage, children swimming, riding bikes, running around laughing, Ken and I relaxing as we watched them play. Now we were waiting for our daughter to have brain surgery. How did we get here?

It was a very surreal time. Victoria appeared to be very healthy aside from the difficulty walking. In fact, as we were walking down the corridor one morning with all our children, another patient's parent asked us, 'Which one of your children is unwell?' Victoria just looked so well. The headaches had subsided.

We were blessed that Victoria was so well. She wasn't hooked up to fluids. She wasn't confined to her bed and the hospital room. We were able to go exploring around the hospital, visiting the various activity rooms and special places for children.

The Fairy Garden was often first on the list to visit each day. It was an outdoor tropical type of garden in the middle of the building. The garden was filled with statues and a couple of cubby houses. Much to the girls' delight, it had fairy costumes to dress up in too.

The Ronald McDonald Family Room was a great place to go when our other children came to visit. There were toys, crafts, books and couches, and movies to watch. It really was set up like a family room you would have at home. The adults could enjoy coffee and a snack in the fenced-off kitchen area. To Ken's pleasure there was a daily newspaper. This was also an excellent place to take other families when they came to visit, away from the confronting oncology ward and hospital rooms.

One of the children's other favourite rooms to visit was the Starlight Express Room. This room was completely geared towards children. It was filled with electronic gaming toys that we didn't have at home. There were always two smiling captains on hand to greet the children as they entered the room, and to get them involved in an activity. Painting was one of the girls' favourite crafts, using as much paint as possible of course.

For us, the favourite room was the Parents' Retreat in the children's oncology ward. It was a room that you needed a special code to get into. No patients or children were allowed, only adults. It was a little haven. I would often retreat to this room to cry, read my Bible, write in my journal and make phone calls.

Ken and I were amazed that all these facilities were available. We quickly began to understand why. Life in hospital can be very trying for both the patient and carers. Our eyes were being opened to a whole new world we hadn't entered voluntarily, but we were determined to make the best of it.

TUESDAY 25TH JANUARY 2011

By Tuesday, we were becoming familiar with the daily hospital routine of meal-times and doctor's rounds. We knew the opening hours of the various activity rooms. Most importantly, we had located all the closest vending machines for midnight snacks.

The play therapist visited Victoria. She was armed with a myriad of craft packs. We were very thankful for these, as they helped pass the time when the activity rooms were closed.

Ken and I met with the neurosurgeon to discuss Victoria's impending surgery. With the help of some knowledgeable friends, I had my list of questions ready for him. It included:

1. Had he been able to consult with other neurosurgeons about the best approach to reach the tumour?

2. If they were not fully confident about performing

the operation here, would they consider transferring Victoria to a larger hospital in Sydney?

3. How long would the surgery take?

4. During the surgery, would someone give us progress reports, and if so, how often?

5. What were the potential side effects of the operation?

As I put this list of questions together, it highlighted what absolute novices we were in this environment. I felt so utterly inadequate. I was very hesitant to even ask these questions, afraid of what the answers would be. Thankfully, my husband did not suffer from the same hesitancy. He just wanted answers. By this time, five days after Victoria's preliminary diagnosis, we had gotten over our initial shock. We were starting to work as a team, drawing on each other's strengths. I would do the research and question writing. Ken would boldly ask the questions. Given so little was known about the tumour, he kept asking until he was satisfied with the answers. Even the length of the operation was unknown, anything from seven to twelve hours. I was glad that God had given me a husband who was able and willing to take a stand for his family when it really mattered.

When Ken asked the questions, I wrote down the doctor's answers as quickly as possible, always trying to capture the exact words he used. I was rapidly learning that doctors chose their words very carefully. Each word spoken had a specific purpose.

Later that morning, we met with the oncologist. We asked the same questions. Thankfully his answers were similar to the neurosurgeon's. While we didn't like some of the answers, such as the worst outcome of surgery would be death, we had confidence that Victoria was in good hands.

Assuming Victoria made it through the surgery, the post operation scenario was very much unknown. After the operation, Victoria would be in the Intensive Care Unit (ICU) for at least twenty-four hours. She would most likely be on a ventilator machine. There was a risk of bleeding in her brain and infection. If there were no post operation complications, she could go home in seven to ten days.

From a physical perspective, it was likely that Victoria would lose her left visual field. The physical weakness on her left side of her body could get worse before it got better, or it could just get worse and be permanent. She could also experience some speech issues.

To get an 'after' picture of Victoria's brain and any possible residual tumour, an MRI was scheduled twenty-four hours post operation. The doctors would use this scan as a baseline to show brain changes in future MRIs.

If the tumour couldn't be completely removed, there were various treatment options, one being more surgery.

Depending on the pathology results, chemotherapy could be used to reduce any residual tumour. Radiation therapy was also an option when Victoria was older. The future was so unclear.

One of our concerns was what do we tell our other children about the operation? We discussed our apprehensions with the oncologist. He gave us two pieces of advice. Firstly, tell them the truth about the operation. Secondly, prepare them for what she will look like after the operation. We had no problems with the second one, 'Next time you see Victoria, her face may look a bit bruised and she will have a bandage around her head.'

The first piece of advice was a bit more challenging. How do you tell a five year old and a seven year old, that their sister may not come home again? Especially when they knew, we had been asking God to heal Victoria. Our children were very aware that something was wrong. Victoria had essentially been in hospital for a week. Our entire extended family was here. Many people had been coming to visit our home. I had signs around the house saying, 'This is big trust God time,' to remind myself of Who was in control.

By the grace of God, we were able to communicate with Marshall and Charlotte the seriousness of the situation. We told them that we were trusting God for the best outcome for Victoria. If that meant Victoria was to go to heaven, then we had to trust that that was the best outcome for her. It mightn't be the best outcome for us, as we would be left here on earth without her, but we had to believe that God had a plan and it was good.

Later that day Ken and I met again with the social worker, who 'prepped' us on what would happen on Thursday, the operation day. We never imagined we would need 'prepping' for such an event. He suggested that we do a tour of the ICU, as Victoria would go there immediately after the operation. The aim of the tour was to familiarise us with the ICU environment and to lessen the shock of potentially seeing Victoria on a ventilator machine.

Our tour began in the ICU waiting room, a big open area complete with kitchen and fridge. While we were looking around the waiting room, I asked the social worker, 'As the surgery is going to take most of the day, would it be all right if I go to the local shopping centre for a couple of hours during the operation?'

He replied something like, 'As the parents, one of you will have to stay on the hospital grounds during the operation, just in case you are needed.'

Now, when I think about that question, I wonder, 'What was I thinking?' How could I even contemplate leaving my three year old daughter while she was having brain surgery? Clearly something in my brain wasn't functioning properly!

When we went into ICU, I understood why visitors were restricted, normally only one visitor at a time. There wasn't a lot of space. Machines were beeping everywhere. The children could come in for a short visit. Either Ken or I could stay with Victoria in ICU on Thursday night after the operation. There was a not-so-comfortable looking fold-out chair to sleep on. The social worker told us that it wouldn't be a restful night with all the machine noises and constant activity.

Our final meeting for the day was with the Nursing Unit Manager (NUM) regarding logistics for Wednesday night and Thursday morning. We got answers to questions such as, when would Victoria need to start fasting in preparation for the operation? Where would we leave our overnight bags while Victoria was in ICU?

It has been a huge day of meetings with doctors and nurses, along with the ICU tour. The enormity of what was about to take place was starting to sink in. We were trying to remain calm about what was ahead and to rest in God's peace. Victoria was well and full of life. She was enjoying all the activities and visitors. The headaches had not returned. With the logistics taken care of, we were looking forward to getting into bed, trusting God would provide us all with a peaceful sleep.

Tomorrow we would celebrate our first Australia Day in hospital.

FAMILY, FUN AND FEAR

WEDNESDAY 26TH JANUARY 2011

Australia Day had arrived. All plans of celebrating on our boat with friends had been shelved. Rather we spent a quiet day moving between Victoria's hospital room and the Ronald McDonald Family Room. A visit from a Delta pet therapy dog was a welcome distraction. We were constantly amazed at the people who volunteered their time, and/or donated money to help families in hospital, whether it was the volunteers in the Ronald McDonald Room, the owners of the Delta Society Dogs or the Starlight Express Room volunteers, just to name of few. All of these precious people made a huge difference to the many hours we spent in hospital.

Various friends dropped in for a visit. I particularly remember a visit from one friend who had her leg in a 'moon' boot. She had hobbled all the way from the carpark at the opposite end of the hospital to the Ronald McDonald Family Room. She gave Victoria a beautiful picture book, 'God knows all about me.' We read that book over and over.

Throughout the day I scribbled thoughts in my notebook. Being a task-focussed, list-making person my thoughts were about all the things I could do while Victoria was in the operating theatre. I was fully in organisation mode. I could easily fill eight to ten hours with activities such as paying our staff, working on the monthly tax return for our business, writing letters to each of the children, reading a few chapters of a book on the significance of birth order, and painting my toenails. Yes, I thought it would be the perfect time to get the toenails in order.

I was making lists, lists and more lists. There was the list of things we would need to take up to ICU, ready for Victoria after the operation. There was another list of things I needed my Mum to bring up to the hospital, including a bag for our dirty washing, which was starting to pile up.

While getting afternoon tea from the staff cafeteria Ken and I saw the neurosurgeon in the hallway. We chatted casually to him, asking if he had had any more thoughts about the approach to the operation. He told us that he hadn't stopped thinking about Victoria since he had met her, and that he felt confident with the route they had decided to take to remove as much of the tumour as possible.

It was a blessing to 'bump' into him, and to hear his heart towards Victoria. We were relieved to have that conversation with him, as we knew we wouldn't see him in the morning before the operation.

Ken and I both stayed at hospital that night. I slept in the room with Victoria. Ken slept in the paediatric palliative care room, which was still vacant. We were hopeful for a peaceful night's sleep so we would all be well-rested for the events of the next day. Peaceful may sound like an odd word to use, but that was how we felt. We had confidence in the surgeon. We had confidence in our daughter's strength of character. But most importantly we had confidence that our God would get us through this, whatever the outcome. And we were exhausted.

As I went to sleep I prayed and meditated on this scripture that a friend who had lost her husband to cancer, had given me. God spoke this word through a prophet to a King and his men who were about to go into battle. He was telling them that He had it all under control and He would be with them.

> *You will not have to fight this battle. Take up your positions; stand firm and see the deliverance the LORD will give you, O Judah and Jerusalem. Do not be afraid; do not be discouraged. Go out and face them tomorrow, and the LORD will be with you.*
> (2 Chronicles 20:17)

This was exactly the encouragement we needed to help us stay positive regarding the physical battle our daughter was going to face in the morning, and for the spiritual battle that we were in. I went to sleep knowing that the LORD was with us. Little did I know that the spiritual battle was about to move to a new level.

It was far from a peaceful night! At 11pm Victoria started to vomit. As the vomiting started, we were reminded of the doctor's words, that vomiting was one of the signs that the tumour was increasing its pressure on the brain. The timing of the surgery was perfect. God's timing was perfect.

Vomiting was a new experience for Victoria. She found it quite fascinating and undertook a detailed study of the food particles in the vomit. 'There's the watermelon mum!' she exclaimed. The nurse came and assisted us in cleaning up Victoria and re-making the bed. Back to sleep we went.

THURSDAY 27TH JANUARY 2011

But not for long - around midnight, Ken received a phone call from the security company that monitor our business premises. They told Ken that the alarm at the office had gone off. Ken and I just looked at each other and laughed. This had never happened before. We knew who was behind it. We knew who was trying to 'rattle our cage'. Was it not enough that Victoria had started to vomit, reminding us of the critical condition of our daughter's health? It appeared not. The devil was still prowling around this time.

> *Be alert and of sober mind. Your enemy the devil prowls around like a roaring lion looking for someone to devour. Resist him, standing firm in the faith, because you know that the family of believers, throughout the world is undergoing the same kind of sufferings.* (1 Peter 5:8-9 NIV)

FAMILY, FUN AND FEAR

We prayed and told the devil to 'get lost in the Name of Jesus.'

Thankfully our business premises were only ten minutes down the road from the hospital, so Ken was able to quickly, in his pyjamas, drive to the office to check out what was going on. When he arrived there, the security guard was there and had assessed the situation. He advised that it was a false alarm. No kidding! Ken safely arrived back at the hospital and we went to bed.

But our much needed restful night's sleep was again cut short by another round of Victoria vomiting at 1.30am. We were once more reminded of the urgency for the need for the surgery. So after another clean-up of Victoria and a change of bed sheets, we literally collapsed into bed around 2.30am, hoping to get four hours sleep straight before having to wake for the operation prep. Victoria was 'nil by mouth' from midnight, needless to say she didn't feel like eating anyway.

Around 7am it was time to take Victoria down to the operating theatre. Ken rode on the bed with Victoria as we went down the long corridor. Victoria thought that was hilarious. All I could do was look around at the people in the corridor going about their daily work, just doing their 'thing'. As I watched and listened, in somewhat of a blur, I was reminded again how quickly the circumstances in life can change. My thoughts were quickly re-focussed on the 'task' at hand, as we arrived in the anaesthetic bay.

Victoria, being compliant as ever, listened attentively to the anaesthetist and following all his instructions, quickly fell 'asleep'. Ken and I gave her a kiss and said, 'See you soon'. What words of faith they were, three simple words, see you soon, but given the enormity of what was about to happen, they carried so much hope. We were hopeful that 'soon' would be sometime later this afternoon, and not the 'soon' of God's timing in heaven.

Once anesthetised, Victoria had another MRI before the operation, to ensure the neurosurgeon had the most up-to-date status of what was happening within her brain.

Ken and I retreated to the cramped small waiting room outside the Operating Theatres. Some of our Christian friends met us there and we took communion, claiming the scripture that it is by Jesus' stripes we are healed.

> *Surely He has borne our griefs (sicknesses, weaknesses, and distresses) and carried our sorrows and pains [of punishment], yet we [ignorantly] considered Him stricken, smitten, and afflicted by God [as if with leprosy]. But He was wounded for our transgressions, He was bruised for our guilt and iniquities; the chastisement [needful to obtain] peace and well-being for us was upon Him, and with the stripes [that wounded] Him we are healed and made whole.*
> (Isaiah 53:4-5)

FAMILY, FUN AND FEAR

We continued to pray together and encourage each other as we waited and waited.

Meanwhile, back on the home front, my sister had taken Charlotte to school. It was Charlotte's first day at kindergarten. And I wasn't there for her. In hindsight, the reality is that I wasn't 'there' for her at all during her first year at school. But that is the sad reality of having a seriously ill child with siblings. As a parent you have to make choices with your time. In this instance the choice really was a 'no brainer' – be with the daughter undergoing brain surgery or be with the daughter starting kindergarten?

The events that are normally considered to be major milestones in a child's life suddenly have lesser significance in a time of crisis, compared to the needs of the seriously ill child. However, as we were to learn later, these choices can have a considerable impact on the siblings. For now, I will just say, I am so grateful for the teachers that took care of Charlotte at school and nurtured her when I couldn't. I am equally grateful for the family, friends and neighbours who encouraged and supported Charlotte throughout that very tumultuous year.

My mum and dad were cleaning up the house and looking after Alexandra. A couple of girl-friends then stepped in to look after Alexandra and the home duties, so mum, dad and my aunt, who had travelled from Wagga Wagga, were free to come up and join us at the hospital. Ken's parents and sister were at the hospital too. It was a day that we all wanted to be together, but didn't know what to say to each other.

By mid-morning, there were quite a few of us at the hospital - so many of us that we quickly out-grew the little waiting room. We were split between the various hospital cafes and the ever peaceful sanctuary of the Ronald McDonald Family Room. There were sufficient people around that Ken and I were quite distracted from the 'main game' happening in the next room.

Around lunch time, while some of us were huddled in the waiting room, the neurosurgeon appeared. We were not expecting to see him until after the operation, so were a little taken aback. He had come out to assure us that all was going well with the operation so far and that a section of the tumour had been sent away for initial pathology. This caring act surprised some of our friends with experience in the medical profession, as the surgeon could have asked someone else to give us an update, but he chose to personally talk to us. We so appreciated his care and concern, as well as his skill and expertise.

My list of activities to fill in the day while we waited remained at the bottom of my bag. How naive I was to even make the list. The chatter and prayer with family and friends were more than sufficient to get through the day.

After eight and a half hours in the operating theatre,

FAMILY, FUN AND FEAR

a nurse came out to advise us that the operation had finished, and that Victoria was sitting up asking for Mummy. No ventilation was required. Hallelujah! The nurse advised us to move down to the ICU waiting room until we were able to see Victoria. We picked up our bags and re-located to a much larger room that included a kitchen.

My recollection is a little sketchy here, but I do remember four things.

1. Eating the cake made by one of our friends.

2. Somehow, I can't actually remember how, finding out that most of the tumour had been removed, and that the initial pathology indicated that the tumour was likely to be a low grade glioma (brain cancer).

3. Then googling on our phones to find out what 'low grade glioma' meant. When we read that low grade probably meant that no more treatment (chemotherapy or radiotherapy) would be required there was another Hallelujah and huge sigh of relief. This of course would need to be confirmed by the oncologist in the days to come.

4. Then phoning and texting family and friends to tell them the news.

It was a time of fervent activity and many, many, many

smiles. Our daughter was still with us and the tumour, as insidious as it was, was not the worst type of tumour. What a day of answered prayers.

- ✓ Reduced time on the operating table, not the predicted ten to twelve hours

- ✓ Victoria still had the ability to speak, no obvious brain damage in that area

- ✓ No ventilation was required, Victoria was able to breathe without intervention

- ✓ No shunt required for increased swelling in her brain

- ✓ Most of the tumour had been removed

- ✓ Initial pathology indicated that the tumour was a low grade glioma

We were soon able to see Victoria in ICU. She appeared to be fine, sleepy, but fine. How wonderful it was to see her breathing without a ventilator, smiling and talking. We really did have so much to be thankful for. Our precious daughter was alive. She was living out her namesake, Victoria, victorious, conqueror; Grace, blessing and favour.

We were so thankful for the steady and skilled hands of the neurosurgeon who removed as much of the tumour as possible without hitting Victoria's brain stem. We were thankful for all the hospital staff that assisted in whatever way, big or small, to make the operation a success. We were thankful for our family and friends who had stood with us on a day that could have had a very different outcome. We were thankful to all the people who prayed for Victoria on that day, and had the faith for a victory. Most of all, we gave thanks to our God who had gone ahead of us and fought the battle.

Only one person was able to stay in ICU with Victoria that night. We decided that I would do the first night, and Ken would do the second night. So Ken went home to see how the other children were doing, especially Charlotte with her first day of kindergarten. We were again grateful to our friends for helping out at home and enabling Ken and me to focus on Victoria's needs.

To say the night in ICU was uncomfortable is an understatement. There was nothing comfortable about the big blue fold-out chair that only partially folded out and had lumps in all the wrong places. The continual necessary observations of Victoria meant much broken sleep for her. For me the beeping machines and staff chatter were finally overcome by a mixture of relief and exhaustion, enabling me to get a few snippets of sleep.

VICTORIA GRACE

REFLECTION - DISTRACTIONS - THERE IS A BATTLE GOING ON

When I think about everything that happened on the night before Victoria's surgery, I am reminded of how the devil attempts to cause havoc in our lives. Havoc designed to distract us from where our focus needs to be – on God.

We continued to rent that office for a further two years, and then another office for a year. Not once in either location, did the alarm go off again. So why did it go off that night? I believe it was meant to rattle Ken and me and shift our focus from God to our circumstances. For seven days Ken and I had been single-mindedly looking to God. We had been working hard to stay in unity, living out of God's promised peace rather than letting the fear and enormity of the situation take over.

When I became a Christian, I bought the book The Spiritual Warrior's Prayer Guide – using God's Word in prayer and spiritual warfare, by Quin Sherrer & Ruthanne Garlock. I devoured it. I read it when I walked to work, memorising scriptures and watching out for cars and other pedestrians at the same time. Here is some of what this book says about spiritual warfare and satan.

> Jesus himself taught his followers a model for prayer which includes this line: "And lead us not into temptation, but deliver us from the evil one" (Matthew 6:13).

In his own great priestly prayer for his followers, Jesus asked the Father to "protect them from the evil one" (John 17:15).

Spiritual warfare is far from a struggle between two near-equal powers, God and satan. We would define it as satan's efforts involving three basic elements:

To destroy the believer's confidence in God and his Son so he or she will forsake the faith.

To seduce them through deceptive teaching or their own sin to believe a lie instead of the truth.

To prevent unbelievers from hearing a clear presentation of the gospel so they will remain in satan's kingdom of darkness.

The devil has real power, which Christians would be wise to respect. But as a created being in no way equal with God, his power is limited. Through the cross, Christ disarmed satan's power and secured victory for the believer who submits to His Lordship (see Colossians 2:15). E.M. Bounds affirms, "To Christ the devil was a very real person. He recognised his personality, felt and acknowledged his power, abhorred his character, and warred against his kingdom. [3]

So here is what I believe was going on that night when the office alarm went off around midnight, on the eve of our daughter's scheduled brain surgery, from which she may have not survived. I believe this alarm was designed to tip us over the edge, to get us to throw our hands up in the air and start to doubt that God was in control. It was a part of a mind game, also having the side-effect of adding to our physical exhaustion.

And then to further challenge our trust in God, the vomiting started. Vomiting was one of the symptoms that we had been told indicates progression of the tumour. I believe the purpose of the vomiting in the mind game was to bring doubt into our minds regarding the timing of the surgery. The onset of the vomiting could have caused us to start panicking, moving into fear that it is too late for surgery and that there is a possibility that Victoria would die before she gets to the operating table.

The enemy was trying to destroy our confidence in God on the very night we needed full confidence in God. We had taken a stand, called people to prayer, had our daughter anointed by the Elders, held an attitude of thankfulness in our hearts, and come together in remarkable calmness and unity. Someone wasn't happy with us. As Joyce Meyer says,

> *The devil never runs out of fiery darts to throw against us when we are trying to go forward. Lift up your shield of faith and remember James*

> *1:2-8 which teaches us that we can ask God for wisdom in trials and He will give it to us and will show us what to do.* [4]

As you have probably gathered from what you've read so far in this book, God's Word is a weapon we continually relied on and trusted in during this journey. His Word brings life, encouragement and peace when we are in the tough places.

Using God's word when you are in the battle is not just about reading the scripture. It is about meditating on it, reading it over and over until it moves from knowledge in your mind, to understanding and then revelation in your heart. Sometimes the process involves reading scripture aloud, making a heartfelt verbal declaration into the atmosphere. Sometimes it involves replacing the pronouns in the verses with your name, or whoever you are praying for. For example, Hebrews 4:16 with my name,

> *Let Wendy approach the throne of grace with confidence, so that Wendy may receive mercy and find grace to help Wendy in her time of need.*

> *In Appendix A I have listed some of the scriptures that we've used over the years when the pressure has come and we've had to make a choice to keep trusting in God despite the circumstances. I pray that they will be a great encouragement to you too.*

Chapter 3

Post Op Recovery

HOSPITAL AND WAITING DAYS

FRIDAY 28TH JANUARY 2011

By 6am I had had enough. I desperately wanted a break. I was just plain worn out. So I phoned home and asked Ken if he could please bring my aunt up to the hospital. I needed someone who had an understanding of the medical world to help me make sense of what was going on after the operation. I knew my aunt would be able to help me, with both her vast nursing experience and her ability to bring calm into a crisis. As soon as I saw her walk in the hospital doors, I felt that a load had lifted. I didn't have to bear these next few hours alone.

Ken sat with Victoria in ICU, allowing my aunt and me time to go down to the staff cafeteria. We sat, ate, talked and cried. Praise God for supportive family – immediate and extended.

Later that morning, Victoria had another MRI to determine how much of the tumour had been removed, and to set a baseline for future MRIs.

After the scan, Victoria returned to ICU and continued to be closely monitored. Ken and I met with the oncologist to discuss the plan going forward. He advised that there was some residual tumour at the brain stem. He also told us that there was swelling around the internal capsule which carries the motor fibres, which was probably why Victoria was not moving her left side. We would not know for a few days whether that lack of movement was temporary, due to the swelling, or permanent, due to a possible loss of blood supply to her brain during the operation. Obviously we were praying for the temporary scenario. Permanent loss would put us on a different journey of suddenly having a child with a physical disability. Physiotherapy would help in the recovery. However she might never recover one hundred percent functionality. So it was still 'wait and see' when it came to how functional Victoria's left side would be.

The oncologist would make a decision on Monday regarding future therapy, but for now the assumption was that no more surgery would be required. He told us that Victoria would be on painkillers for two or three days. She would be on an IV for fluids and her fluid output would be closely monitored for fluid retention.

After this meeting, Ken left the hospital and returned to work. Unfortunately, having just made it through the Global Financial Crisis, our business was not in the position to afford him the luxury of paid annual leave. His business responsibilities needed to be attended to alongside family responsibilities. It was extremely tough for Ken to bear the financial pressure along with the deep concern for his daughter's well-being. However, at least work provided some sort of distraction.

When I arrived back in ICU to be with Victoria, she was pointing to her leg. 'Touch my leg,' she said.

I touched her leg, and then immediately she spoke again, 'No, touch my arm.'

So I touched her arm. Then, again, instantly, she said, 'No, not there, touch my tummy,' her speech getting more and more frantic.

Victoria repeated this behaviour for an hour or so, to the point of becoming inconsolable. We prayed. Nothing changed. We asked the staff if they had a DVD player or TV. The nursing staff wheeled in an antiquated VCR machine with a library of children's videos. I asked Victoria what she wanted to watch, she replied, 'Bob the Builder.'

So we put on Bob the Builder, hoping that would bring some peace into the room. But no, it didn't. Almost immediately Victoria said, 'No, I want to watch Thomas now,' pointing to another video on the trolley.

We changed the video, and again within seconds,

Victoria's response was, 'No, I want that one,' pointing to yet another video on the trolley.

This indecision and irritability continued for another hour or so. This behaviour was so out of character for Victoria. Her erratic demanding was starting to cause a disturbance in ICU. So much so, that the nurse assigned to the patient in the next room came into Victoria's room and not-so-politely said, 'Could you tell your child to be better behaved?'

This request tipped me over the edge. I had been holding my emotions together quite well until this time. I just lost it and snapped loudly, 'This is one of the most well behaved children you could ever meet, but right now she is very unwell. Can you leave this room now! '

I know I wasn't polite. I was incensed at the nurse's complete lack of understanding of the situation. We weren't in a normal ward. We were in ICU. Our daughter was critically ill. I think expecting good behaviour was completely unrealistic. In all our years of hospital stays and visits, that is the one and only time we have had an interaction with a less than understanding medical professional. It prompted me to suggest in the feedback survey that the hospital needed an Intensive Care Unit for children, separate from adult patients, complete with paediatric trained staff.

Throughout the day Victoria continued to get more and

more irritable. Thankfully Ken returned to the hospital mid-afternoon so I could get to school in time to pick up Marshall and Charlotte. At least I made it to Charlotte's second day in kindergarten. Just quietly, I was very glad I was going home and that Ken was going to do the night shift. I was struggling with Victoria's behaviour. Fear was starting to set in. What was going on in her brain?

As I drove to the school I felt myself becoming more and more anxious about Victoria and her state of mind. Yesterday after the operation she had seemed so calm and 'normal'. Today she was like a completely different child whose brain was scrambled, unable to decide what she wanted, erratic in her speech, agitated with anyone who came near her. During the surgery they needed to retract the temporal lobe which processes memory which could have been making her very confused. What would that mean for her in the long term?

To help ease my anxiety I played some worship music. As I drove listening to the music, I felt the Holy Spirit speak to me, 'It's okay. It's just the drugs that she is on for the pain.'

Immediately after hearing those words I felt a peace in my heart. Victoria was going to be okay. With that reassurance I was able to go to school with a smile on my face, albeit a very tired face.

First stop at school was Charlotte's class room. I can still remember walking into the classroom and breathing with relief when I saw her teacher, knowing that she was in such capable loving hands: Knowing too, that Charlotte would be well looked after at school, a place of security and stability, when our home environment was so chaotic.

Marshall was waiting with Charlotte, already assuming the big brother role with so much maturity at such a young age. They were just as delighted to see me as I was to see them. It was hugs all round.

'How is Victoria? Is she home?' they asked in unison.

We walked to the car, chatting about their day at school. How nice it was to be doing something 'normal' again, and to be out of the intense hospital environment. Although I couldn't quite bring myself to do the smile and wave thing to the other school mums, at least I was physically there for Marshall and Charlotte. The three of us continued to chat the whole way home.

When we arrived home, I quickly said my hellos to family and friends, and went directly to my computer. There was something I knew I just had to do – new signs. I sat down and made some new ones to go around our home. They said, 'This is a PRAISE God time'. I have since gained the understanding that God asks us to praise Him no matter what circumstance in which we find ourselves. I printed and laminated the signs and displayed them in various rooms, including outside our front door. After I had made this visible declaration of God's goodness, I was able to sit down out the back with family and friends. I could take a breath and talk about the wonders of the past seven days and how good our God had been to our family.

About 8pm Ken phoned from the hospital to say the doctor had decided to move Victoria from ICU, down to the paediatric oncology ward. The nurses were going to turn off the morphine, as that was probably the cause of the agitation and itchiness. They would try an alternative pain relief. I said a quiet prayer.

'Thank you Holy Spirit, you knew exactly what was going on and you told me.'

SATURDAY 29TH JANUARY 2011

Mid-morning I arrived at the hospital to swap shifts with Ken. I was so grateful to have had a peaceful night's sleep at home. Conversely, Ken was very keen to go home and get some of that peaceful sleep.

Victoria's room was again directly behind the nurses' station so if anything went wrong, she could quickly be attended to. She was looking well, although her right eye was shut and puffy.

Once I had unpacked, the nurse debriefed me on the night's activities. She informed me that when the morphine was turned off, the itchiness had stopped and Victoria had slept for four hours. Other pieces of critical information she relayed to me were that Victoria had done two wees and eaten two little tubs of ice-cream.

Within herself Victoria seemed so much calmer, a bit grumpy, but nowhere near as irritated and confused as she was yesterday. She was able to have a coherent conversation, and knew exactly where she was. What a different child to the one I had left in the hospital yesterday afternoon. We were so grateful that the pain medication issue had been resolved. She was now on Oxycodeine and Panadol.

The generosity of people and organisations continued to amaze us. There was an elderly couple who made patchwork quilts that cleverly converted into pillows for the children in hospital. The quilts added some vibrant colour to any white sterile rooms. Knitted toys were freely given away each time we went to the Ronald McDonald Family Room. Captain Starlight had visited Victoria in ICU and presented her with a bag full of gifts. These toys and gifts helped Victoria, and her visiting siblings, to pass the time.

SUNDAY 30TH JANUARY 2011

Nothing spectacular about this day, other than our daughter was living and breathing. Praise God! We just hung out in the J1 ward at John Hunter Hospital, making good use of all the activity bags, crafts and books. Victoria continued on the pain medication, with close supervision from the nurses.

POST OP RECOVERY

MONDAY 31ST JANUARY 2011

It was hair washing day, so off to the bath we went. The bath was one of the highlights in J1. It was huge. You could raise the entire bath up and down. Turning the water on and off was done via buttons. Hair washing was a very tricky 'operation' as we tried not to wet the wound site which ran from the middle of Victoria's forehead along her hair line to behind her right ear.

Later in the day we met with the neurosurgeon. He explained that during the operation he had found that the tumour became less distinct the closer he got to the brain stem. His impression from the post operation MRI was that the tumour probably arose from the brain stem.

A friend with knowledge in this area has since told me, 'The art of neurosurgery is knowing when to stop.'

Thankfully the neurosurgeon operating on Victoria knew when to stop. He advised us that the key things to watch for now were infection under the bone or swelling. Thankfully, Victoria was still in the room behind the nurses' station, so they could keep a very close eye on her.

She was eating and drinking by herself. The pain medication was now being given orally rather than intravenously. Having the drip removed from Victoria's hand was a relief. It had been a little tricky getting her to the toilet, carrying her in one arm, and walking the drip pole and pump in the other hand.

The neurosurgeon encouraged Victoria to try walking and weight bearing on her left leg. He said a physiotherapist would visit us on the ward to make a therapy plan for home. Most of the therapy would be play based.

Finally, when we asked about the timeframe for leaving hospital, he said it was dependent on a couple of things, including Victoria doing a poo. She was doing plenty of wees, but we had yet to see a poo. The pain medication was making her constipated. Getting her to poo became our focus.

> *From this point forward in our journey, I started communicating with family and friends via email. This mass communication method enabled me to provide a single update on Victoria's well-being to many people, instead of fielding multiple phone calls. It reduced the emotional drain of having to continually explain Victoria's current status. The emails also enabled me to communicate specific prayer requests for her.*

POST OP RECOVERY

EMAIL SENT ON 31ST JANUARY 2011

Thank you so much for your prayers for Victoria Grace and our family. Her progress since the eight hour operation last Thursday has been amazing. Understandably Victoria has been very grumpy since waking from the operation, giving plenty of orders to us, the nursing staff and doctors. At least we know that her speech has not been impacted by the operation.

However today, when she saw Alexandra for the first time since the operation Victoria's face lit up, smiling and laughing, wanting her sister to sit in bed with her and play blocks. To see her returning to her normal beautiful disposition brought joy to our hearts.

And to top that off, when we went into the Ronald McDonald family room, Victoria started standing and walking by herself, albeit slowly and a bit wobbly. Again there were some tears in our eyes. Then we ventured out to the play area, and with a bit of assistance she climbed the steps on the play equipment and went down the slide.

Praise God for such a speedy recovery. Please continue to pray for a smooth recovery, with no infections or bleeding, and continuing strengthening of Victoria's left side.

Within the next day or so we will meet with the oncologist and find out whether further treatment is required.

Thank you again for your prayers, love and support. We know we are definitely not alone on this journey.

EMAIL SENT ON 1ST FEBRUARY 2011

We have spoken with both Victoria's surgeon and oncologist today.

The surgeon is hopeful that she will be able to go home by the end of the week due to the way the recovery is going. This is great news, as even though our hospital experience has been very positive, home is where we all really want to be. We had a great time with the music therapist this afternoon. All the children were at the hospital joining in the fun; the therapist was a little overwhelmed and thought we should ask for a bigger room.

The oncologist said the tumour was a low grade glioma. This is good news too. The exact type of low grade tumour is still to be determined, a second pathology opinion is being sought and we should know the exact type, at the earliest, early next week.

Depending on the pathology outcome, the treatment will be either an MRI every three months or chemotherapy for a period of time.

Please continue to uphold Victoria in your prayers, that her recovery will continue to go well, and that she will get confidence to use her left arm and hand again. She is currently not really using them, favouring the right hand and arm. Her walking is improving each day. Tomorrow we will meet with the physio and occupational therapist to develop a program for her.

Thank you again for your continued prayers and support.

EMAIL SENT ON 3RD FEBRUARY 2011

The last two days have been charged with emotion. I think the enormity of what we have just been through, and uncertainty of the future, has become a reality and we are slowly coming out of the 'state of shock' we have been in.

Victoria herself is coming along well. We had a good session with the physiotherapist and occupational therapist this morning, learning how to encourage movement through play. The immediate goal with walking is to get Victoria to put weight on her left leg and therefore put her foot flat on the floor, rather than walking on tippee toes. They made a delightful red boot for her to wear at night time to stretch out the foot. Regarding the left arm and hand, she now has a little glove to help strengthen her wrist and encourage her fingers to stretch out. There is a lot to learn for all of us!

Unfortunately the family support team at home were struck down with vomiting and diarrhoea on Tuesday night, so they were unable to visit us until late today. As a result Victoria and I have practically been in quarantine, with Victoria unable to leave her hospital room, as we are in a ward with other children having chemotherapy with low or no immunity. Another little challenge for us.

Finally it looks as though we can go home tomorrow, as long as Victoria does a poo. So please put that on your prayer list for tonight, thanks.

A friend emailed me these scriptures this afternoon, so timely and a reminder that the strength we need for this time will come from God alone.

For Victoria's left side healing,

> *He gives power to the weak, and to those who have no might he increases strength.* (Isaiah 40:29 NKJV)

For the Robinsons,

> *But they that wait upon the Lord shall renew their strength; they shall mount up with wings as eagles, they shall run, and not be weary, they shall walk and not faint.* (Isaiah 40:31 NIV)

Please continue to uphold Victoria and our family in your prayers as we continue to trust God at this time.

> *If you are interested in a few more details about Victoria's medical diagnosis (brain cancer and acquired hemiplegia), Appendix B – Victoria's medical diagnoses - has some further definitions and explanations.*

REFLECTION - THE HOLY SPIRIT – OUR COMFORTER

As you have just read in this chapter, when I left the hospital on the Friday afternoon after Victoria's operation, my concern for Victoria's well-being was growing; fear and anxiety were beginning to take hold. In this reflection I am going to revisit this event in a bit more detail as it is a great example of how the Holy Spirit can bring truth into a circumstance and therefore peace into our hearts.

The day after the brain surgery Victoria was acting very differently to the child we knew her to be. It was as if some major rewiring had taken place in her brain. My heart began to grow heavy with questions like, 'What if this is how she is going to be now?' I was crying out to God, 'What is going on? Is she going to be okay?'

Thankfully in the fifteen years of being a Christian, I had learnt that worshipping God is one of the best things to do when anxiety surfaces and fearful thoughts try to take hold. The decision to put some worship music on during that drive home from the hospital, enabled me to change my focus on the fearful thoughts, to thoughts of Who my Heavenly Father is, and all I have to be thankful for. I can't even remember what worship songs I was listening too. But I can remember tears streaming down my face as I wrestled with how I had seen our daughter acting in the hospital. I was desperate to know what was going on.

It was in that place of desperation, combined with a deep

cry for mercy and understanding that I heard the still small voice of the Holy Spirit say to me, 'It's okay. It's just the drugs that she is on for the pain.'

Hearing those words, the truth of the situation, gave me peace. I knew then, that how I had seen our daughter behaving was only temporary. Later that evening, Ken's phone call confirmed that. He phoned from the hospital and said that the morphine had been causing the agitation and itchiness. The doctors were going to give Victoria alternative pain relief.

Without that insight from the Holy Spirit, I could have spent five hours allowing myself to become more and more anxious about a situation that was going to be resolved. I would have been completely inattentive to our other children and definitely unable to sit with family and friends at home, and declare how good God had been to our family.

But because of the insight the Holy Spirit had given me, I was able to connect, even if only in a limited way with Marshall and Charlotte. I was able to praise God wholeheartedly, and celebrate with family and friends.

I realise that for some people reading this book you may not have heard of the Holy Spirit before. Or if you have, maybe do not know much about Him and the blessing He wants to be in your life. I am not a theological scholar, but I know from my experience that the Holy Spirit is real, and an essential part of God's plan to transform us to be more like Christ. For completeness I have included some theological information about the Holy Spirit from David Cartledge.

> *The Doctrine of the Holy Spirit is of great importance judging from the place He occupies in the Holy Scriptures. With the exception of 2nd & 3rd John every book in the New Testament contains a reference to the Spirit's work. The Holy Spirit is a person, not an influence or power of God, not an ethereal substance diffused through space, not the impulses to righteousness that come to men.*
>
> *He is the third person of the Trinity, the executor of the Godhead. He is seen in the act of creation, empowering men for service, communicating to men the revelation of God and so directing them to record God's truth without error.* [5]

The Holy Spirit is always with us. He will give us insight, if we ask Him and make space in our myriad of thoughts to listen to Him. The Holy Spirit, our Comforter, who Jesus said would come after Him, to teach us all things:

> *But the Comforter (Counselor, Helper, Intercessor, Advocate, Strengthener, Standby), the Holy Spirit, Whom the Father will send in My name [in My place, to represent me and act on My*

behalf], He will teach you all things. And He will cause you to recall (will remind you of, bring to your remembrance) everything I have told you. Peace I leave with you; My [own] peace I now give and bequeath to you. Not as the world gives do I give to you. Do not let your hearts be troubled, neither let them be afraid. [Stop allowing yourselves to be agitated and disturbed; and do not permit yourselves to be fearful and intimidated and cowardly and unsettled.] (John 14:26-27)

In the past fifteen years, God had not only been teaching me about the importance of worship for developing a more intimate relationship with Him, He had also been teaching me about His Holy Spirit and what He can do in my life if I yield to Him. Charles R. Swindoll explains it this way,

He longs to empower us with His dynamic presence, change our attitudes, warm our hearts, show us how and where to walk, comfort us in our struggles and our sorrows, strengthen us in the weak and fragile places of our lives, and literally revolutionise our pilgrimage from this planet to paradise. [6]

In any relationship, greater intimacy takes time to develop. Our relationship with the Holy Spirit is no different. It takes time and a willingness to be vulnerable and allow the Holy Spirit to guide us.

In practical terms I have found this means surrendering each day to God. Literally saying to Him, 'I lay down my plans for today, may Your will be done.' Then, with situations that happen throughout the day, praying, often in tongues, my heavenly language, asking the Holy Spirit for wisdom, a word of direction or comfort.

In my experience He has never failed to provide that insight, as long as I remember to ask for it. And that is one of the keys, not to get tied up in my own thoughts and knowledge, but rather to continually seek the Holy Spirit's wisdom and discernment.

To conclude this reflection, here is another example of how the Holy Spirit has helped me. About six months after Victoria was diagnosed our family found itself in crisis mode again, due to the illness of another family member. Things were in absolute turmoil and I had the responsibility of determining what would be best for our family at that time. I was in the shower that morning, talking to the Holy Spirit, asking for His guidance. Specifically I needed the right words to say in a phone conversation that was going to take place later that day. The well-being of our family was dependent on a good outcome from that phone call. I felt the Holy Spirit give me the exact phrase to use in that conversation.

Later that morning, during the phone call, and the

conversation wasn't going particularly well. There appeared to be a lack of understanding of what our family required. It was at that time that I felt prompted to speak the phrase the Holy Spirit had given me. Immediately the whole tone of the conversation changed. It was like there was a sudden revelation on the other end of the phone about what action needed to be taken. We were in complete agreement.

That one conversation led to decisions that over the years have enabled our family to be restored physically, emotionally and spiritually. Only the Holy Spirit would have known what needed to be said then, to bring to pass what was needed for the future years.

My prayer is that after reading these testimonies of what can happen when you allow the Holy Spirit to speak into your life, you will be encouraged to yield and live a life more open to His guidance.

> *But I say, walk and live [habitually] in the [Holy] Spirit [responsive to and controlled by the Spirit]; then you will certainly not gratify the cravings and desires of the flesh (of human nature without God).* (Galatians 5:16)

Chapter 4

Home and Rehabilitation

EMAILS FROM 8TH FEB TO 3RD MAR 2011

EMAIL SENT ON 8TH FEBRUARY 2011

Well, we have been at home for four full days now, and full they have been. The home is back to running as 'normally' as it can, with the ever helpful hands of my mother, Granny Bett.

Victoria is walking better each day, gaining more and more strength in her left leg. The little cherry red ankle boots are helping heaps. Today I have even noticed her, a couple of times, standing flat footed with her weight evenly distributed on both legs. Prior to this she would always lean noticeably to the right-hand side. So that is good progress, for which we thank God. The Occupational Therapist (OT) we saw at the hospital today, was very impressed with her improved walking too.

We have been doing the exercises with the left hand and wrist each day, accompanied by singing nursery rhymes. Victoria is very amenable to doing the exercises, again her personality and determination coming to the fore. I was amused however, to see her playing with her doll, and saying to the doll, 'come on, sit down here, now give me your hand so we can do your exercises'.

The session with the OT today was fruitful, giving us lots of ideas for different styles of play that will help Victoria start to use her left hand more, and in the correct way. Although I must say it was quite overwhelming to see just how little she can actually do with her hand at present. Even picking up a wooden block was very difficult for her, requiring intense concentration, of which she is capable, we thank God again that that part of her brain is unaffected. The tears did start to come to my eyes as I began to get more of an appreciation of the journey we are just beginning.

However, by the end of the day, I had been reminded once again, in a very tangible way, that we are not on this journey alone, and that our loving heavenly father will provide all that we need.... On the way home from the hospital I was saying to mum that I didn't think that I would be able to take Victoria and Alexandra weekly to the hospital for the OT and physio by myself, both from a practical and emotional perspective, and I would need to get some sort of roster going with friends, neighbours etc. to help me. And guess what, by the end of the day I had bumped into a neighbour at the shopping centre who said, 'I can't cook, is there anything else I can do for you? Secondly, I had a message on my answer phone from another neighbour saying, how can we help? Thirdly, another neighbour came to our front gate asking how they could help us. So there are three people already on the roster.

Thank you again for your prayers and support, we pray we will continue to see Victoria's strength, gross and fine motor skills develop fully.

EMAIL SENT ON 12TH FEBRUARY 2011

What can I say? We have an amazing God and a determined daughter. Our physio and OT appointment on Thursday was very positive. They could not believe that Victoria could now voluntarily turn her left hand palm from facing up to facing down, and they were equally amazed at her improved walking balance. The exact words of the physio regarding the arm/hand movement, were 'the messages are definitely getting through from the brain to the arm and hand' - Praise God.

There is still a lot of improvement to come, but it is awesome for both Victoria and us to see the progress made to date. Victoria is now including her left hand more often in play rather than ignoring it completely. She has great delight in showing us how she can make the diamond with both hands while singing 'Twinkle Twinkle Little Star' - something that used to be so simple for her to do, but now requires intense concentration. Please continue to pray for a full recovery of left side gross and fine motor skills.

On Monday we will see the oncologist and find out if further treatment is required. Please pray that God will give us all the strength to cope regardless of the treatment required.

Thank you again for your prayers and support.

EMAIL SENT ON 14TH FEBRUARY 2011

We trekked up to the hospital this morning, only to find out that the second opinion on the pathology had not yet arrived. This was disappointing.

However, the Oncologist did advise that he thought it was most likely that the second opinion would agree with his diagnosis that Victoria's treatment in relation to the tumour would be an MRI every three months for two years, and then every six months for another two years and then probably one scan every year until doctors determine otherwise. This is a very positive outcome.

If the residual tumour, 11 mm at the brain stem, did start to grow in the future, depending on the location of the growth, either more surgery or chemotherapy would be the likely treatment. The regular MRIs would provide an indication of growth. We pray that Victoria will not need to face either of these situations in the future.

So for now we just need to keep waiting for the results, praying and doing exercises. Hopefully we will have a definitive answer regarding treatment by the end of the week.

Victoria within herself is absolutely fantastic. She is enjoying getting out on the tricycle, with Granny Bett doing quite a bit of pushing. Concerts are still a favourite activity, with varying instruments including bells, tambourine, mini guitar and even a bit of piano. We have an OT appointment on Wednesday and then a combined OT/Physio appointment on Friday. We sadly have to say good bye to Granny Bett on Thursday.

Thanks again for your support and prayers, both are invaluable to us all. We know our God is in control, in Him we trust.

EMAIL SENT ON 22ND FEBRUARY 2011

As I write this email I am watching the devastation caused in Christchurch by the earthquake and what do you say? Nothing to do except pray.

As for our beautiful Victoria, we don't have much to report at the moment.

Our last two hospital visits have been cancelled due to a sick doctor and an OT with family sickness.

We are still waiting on the second opinion from the pathologist ….

At the physio/OT session last Friday, both therapists thought Victoria's improvement with both her walking and arm/hand movements were 'fantastic' so that was hugely encouraging.

At home Victoria is voluntarily using her left hand more and more in everyday activities, for example, dressing herself, carrying plates from the table, puzzle play and carrying toys around.

Most of the stitches on her head have dissolved, there are only about seven left visible. We have a follow-up appointment with the neurosurgeon next week, and hopefully he will give her the okay to go swimming again.

A couple of people have asked me about the impact of this event on the other children. Well, here is a window into the world of Charlotte.

Last Friday we had been home from hospital after therapy for about half an hour, when I received a call from the school to say that Charlotte had been coughing all morning, and could I come and pick her up as they were concerned that she could have whooping cough, which had been going around. So I went and picked up Charlotte and took her to our GP. The GP checked out Charlotte and looked at me as to say, 'why have you brought your child here?' Note; there had been no coughing since we had left school. The GP suggested we should stay away from other people until the coughing ceased.

HOME AND REHABILITATION

By bed-time on Friday night, there had still been no coughing so I asked Charlotte how the cough was, and she replied, "I don't think I will have the cough at the weekend mummy, but it will probably come back on Monday."

Needless to say Charlotte received a lot of love and re-assurance over the weekend. Thanks again for the prayers and support.

EMAIL SENT ON 2ND MARCH 2011

We had a very good meeting with Victoria's neurosurgeon this morning. He said Victoria's scar had healed well and she could go swimming again. This is good news as Victoria can now start hydrotherapy next week. He was also impressed with the amount of strength Victoria had re-gained to date in her left hand. We will next see him a week after the MRI scan scheduled for 5th May. Hopefully the scan will show no change in the residual tumour.

We are still waiting for the second opinion to return regarding the tumour. The neurosurgeon assured us once again that it was not time-critical to get these results back.

Tomorrow we will be up to the hospital again for another OT/Physio session. The OT has made a splint for Victoria to wear on her hand at night to help the fingers extend out, so the brain can start to get the message that 'extension' is a normal position for the fingers. Victoria continues to be ever so compliant at night, wearing both her half leg cast and now the hand splint.

The OT has also made a puppet glove for Victoria's right hand; we decorated it with eyes, hair and a face. When we are doing puzzles or the Tupperware shape ball at home, Victoria wears the puppet glove as a reminder that the right hand is not to help the left hand with its tasks. Again, she is very compliant and the glove adds a little humour to the exercises.

Thank you again for your prayer support. We know that this great recovery we are witnessing is a direct answer to prayer.

EMAIL SENT ON 3RD MARCH 2011

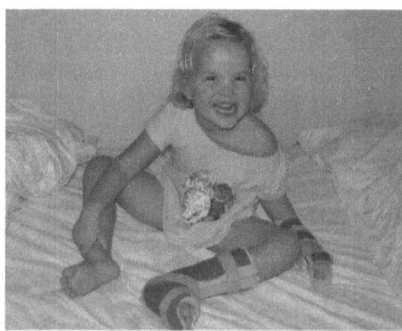

Victoria at home wearing the night boot and arm splint

It is Thursday 3rd March, five weeks exactly since Victoria Grace came out of eight and half hours of surgery. The attached photo, with her wearing her night time splints to stop her leg muscles contracting, sums up Victoria's attitude during this whole journey. She is one truly amazing girl.

Today we finally got the results of the second opinion on the tumour – it was the same as the original results – so the only treatment required will be the three monthly scans for two years and subsequent scans. The relief that we felt when we got this confirmation was huge, which really is an understatement!

We had a very good session with the OT this morning. They videoed Victoria to get a 'baseline' of her current ability with her left arm, hand and fingers, so it will be interesting to watch it again in a few months' time, when even more progress has been made.

A friend and I were praying this afternoon, and the verse that was in my journal was...

> *It is good to give thanks to the Lord, and to sing praises to Your name, O Most High; To declare Your lovingkindness in the morning, and Your faithfulness every night.* (Psalm 92:1-2 NIV)

What more is there to say????

Thanks again for your prayer and practical support. Love Ken, Wendy and family.

PS: for anyone who is interested, here is my list of reasons, some big and some practical, not in any particular order, I wrote on the 22nd January, three days after the tumour was discovered, to thank God for in relation to the timing of the discovery of the tumour:

1. Midwife Friend – detection of the something seriously wrong with Victoria, wisdom and grace.

2. Doctor Friend – wisdom and grace.

3. Friend – friendship and availability to stay with the children the night I took Victoria to the emergency department.

4. Family – unconditional love and support.

5. Employee – new sales rep in Melbourne that Ken employed the day after the tumour was discovered.

6. Photoboards of family events that I had created just after Christmas and were hanging in the kitchen, something I hadn't ever done before.

7. Mum – her new passport returned the day before the tumor was detected.

8. Victoria – healthy, no pain and able to do most things.

9. My sister and family – here in Australia, holidaying at Byron Bay, at the time the tumour was detected.

10. Muffins for school morning tea and lunches were cooked and in the freezer.

11. Friend's email from Rick Warren about life being a set of railway tracks – experiencing the good and the bad at the same time.

12. Marshall's 2011 teacher is an 'emailing' teacher who had already made contact with us parents via email.

13. I had just bought a lot of plastic containers to store food.

14. Church family – wonderful support.

15. Neighbours – wonderful support.

16. Business – Our staff manager, able to keep the office running without need for Ken's involvement.

17. Business – financial turnaround in the past 6 months.

18. Ken – openness and willingness to show his emotions, not suppress them. The social worker at the hospital said that he had never met another man who was so open with his emotions as Ken is.

19. Marriage counselling we have done over the years which helped Ken and I to really understand each other.

20. Prayer girls – a group of girls that I'd meet regularly with to pray about things going on in our lives and our family's lives.

21. Summertime.

22. I had finished breastfeeding Alexandra.

23. All the school preparations (uniforms etc) done.

HOME AND REHABILITATION

REFLECTION – REHAB – CONQUERING AND CREATIVITY

With our first three children we decided to wait until they were born to find out their sex, however when I was pregnant with our fourth child, Marshall, aged six at the time, was very keen to have a brother. So at the twenty week scan we found out the baby's sex. Marshall was getting another sister. Thankfully he had another twenty weeks to get used to the idea.

Anyway, as we didn't know the sex of the first three children while I was pregnant, Ken and I agreed that he would choose a boy's name and I a girl's name. When I was seeking God for a girl's name for our third child, He responded with the name Victoria Grace. Victoria, being the feminine form of the name Victor, is Latin for victory or conquer. Grace, derived from the Latin 'gratia', meaning God's favour. What a name – Victory, conquer, God's favour.

A couple of months before I gave birth, we were in church, standing during worship. At the end of the worship time, the pastor said he felt we were all to shout out 'Victorious'. So being an obedient congregation we did. Over and over again, the word Victorious was shouted out into the atmosphere. In among the shouting, I heard that still small voice again, confirming, 'This is the name of your child.'

In October, we were blessed with a baby girl, whom we of course named, Victoria Grace. Just over three years later, as she lay on the bed of the CT scanner at midnight, I felt God remind me that she has all that she needs to deal with this. She is a victor, a conqueror and she has God's favour on her.

As the years have gone by I have realised more and more, just how anointed she is for this journey, a journey that most definitely requires a conquering spirit.

> *Yet amid all these things we are more than conquerors and gain a surpassing victory through Him Who loved us.* (Romans 8:37)

Again and again we have witnessed this conquering spirit rise up and enable her to valiantly take on whatever challenge she is facing. For example, a daily stretching and exercise routine for a three year old is a big ask. However, the determination she has shown has meant that the functionality in her left leg, arm and hand has not only been maintained, but over the years it slowly keeps improving.

This determination has been complimented by a positive and grateful attitude we have worked hard to instil in our children. An attitude that says, 'Hey, some things in my life aren't great right now, but I do have many things to be thankful for' - an attitude that focuses on what God has to say about us and our lives. Joyce Meyer, in her book, Battlefield of the Mind says,

> *God has a perfect plan for each of us, and we can't control Him with our thoughts and words. But, we must think and speak in agreement with His will and plan for us. If you don't have any idea what God's will is for you at this point, at least begin by thinking, "Well, I don't know God's plan, but I know He loves me. Whatever He does will be good, and I'll be blessed."*
>
> *Begin to think positively about your life. Practice being positive in each situation that arises. Even if whatever is taking place in your life at the moment is not good, expect God to bring good out of it, as He has promised in His word.* [7]

An immense amount of organisation and creativity combined with Victoria's conquering spirit, helped to keep her regular physical therapy sessions from becoming too onerous. It is critical that the therapy is continued in some way throughout her life, as lack of use of muscle groups could mean that any functional gains made during the early years are lost. The transition between the pre-school therapy programs and commencing school is a time when parents especially need to advocate and seek out the support their child needs. An organisation supporting children with hemiplegia in the UK, Hemihelp, found that,

Almost half of the Hemihelp parent members who filled in our survey form were not satisfied with the frequency of the therapy their child received, especially after reaching school age. [8]

Here are some of the strategies I have used over the past five plus years to maintain this frequent daily exercise regime, and maintain my sanity, no joke. Later on in the book I share some of the creative strategies we have used to add variety and fun to the regime.

Ask for help. Don't try to do it all yourself.

As the mum, or primary carer we can so often try to do everything ourselves. But that approach, in my experience, leads to a very cranky, resentful mum/carer. I have also found that there are many kind people around who have the time, knowledge and desire to help out. We just need to ask for help. For example, when Victoria was doing a two week home-based intensive occupational therapy program, I had a roster of volunteers, neighbours, school teachers and church friends, who helped either with the therapy or with looking after our other children.

Seek out funding from both government and non-government programs.

There are funding programs available to help families with children with disabilities. It just takes time and a lot of emotional energy to advocate for your child to ensure they get the support they need. But again, to help maintain your sanity as the primary carer, I believe it's absolutely necessary to access this assistance. On occasions we have received funding for a therapy support person to come to our home during the week to help Victoria with her stretching and exercise program. This practical support has made a huge difference to me. Our afternoons were already busy with four sets of homework, extra-curricular activities and preparing dinner, so finding the time to fit in Victoria's hour of physical therapy was a huge challenge.

Give your child some control over what happens in the therapy session.

When the therapy is on-going year after year, it can be difficult to keep the child engaged and focused. Creativity plays a huge part in continuing engagement. So does giving your child an element of control, particularly as the child matures and grows in their understanding of why the therapy is necessary. As they get older the child may become more aware of the physical consequences of not doing the therapy. In Victoria's case, it makes no real difference to me or the therapist if she doesn't do the exercises. However for her, if she doesn't do them it means pain in her legs, reduced mobility and reduced ability to do two handed activities. So we give her some control by allowing her to select the specific exercises for each muscle group and choose the order in which the exercises will be done. This helps her to feel that she isn't being 'told' what to do all the time. She is empowered

Get equipped.

Having some equipment on hand for therapy sessions is definitely advantageous. At home we have a creativity box filled with activities to help develop fine motor skills. Each session Victoria chooses an activity from that box. The contents of the box have changed over the years from playdough, to modelling clay, threading buttons to beading, wooden puzzles to mind puzzles like the Rubik's cube. We also have some equipment outside, ready to assist with developing gross motor skills. Victoria has access to these boxes both during assigned therapy times, and in general play. We are always listening out for activities she is talking about, to see whether in some way, overtly or subtly, we can introduce them into our daily life. For example, at one time there was a lot of chatter about loombands. They are miniature rubber bands that can be knotted together to make bracelets, necklaces and other creative forms. Loombands are perfect for developing fine motor skills, and most importantly they weren't viewed as therapy because everyone else at school was doing them too.

Involve the siblings.

Often when one sibling has special needs the other siblings can feel left out and neglected, even though that is not the parents' intention. For example, if one of your children has quality time as their primary love language, these times of crisis are not going to work well for them, as mum does not have a lot of quality time to give. I have found that by involving the other siblings whenever possible in these therapy sessions, it builds a greater sense of family, as well as developing skills and empathy. This involvement has either been in the planning of the therapy, working alongside Victoria in the therapy sessions, or joining in the celebrations when the therapy is finished. All equally important aspects of the process.

Build good relationships with therapists.

Throughout Victoria's rehabilitation we have been blessed with extremely professional and skilled therapists. They have done an incredible job with a lot of patience. My suggestion to all parents is to continually show your appreciation to all therapists involved with your children, especially with regular words of encouragement about the difference they are making in your child's life. I also believe it is important to encourage your child to show their appreciation too, with manners and small homemade gifts when appropriate.

Watch, listen and learn at therapy sessions.

While sometimes it is tempting to think that one therapy session a week, or month is sufficient to maintain or improve your child's well-being, the reality is that normally it isn't. Most often the therapy needs to be done daily or at least every two days for a period of time, or it may be on-going. Ultimately your young child is your responsibility. I have learnt that I need to understand all the ins and outs of the therapy sessions, so that whenever an opportunity presents itself in everyday life, we can implement some aspect of the therapy either overtly or covertly. For example, overtly, when Victoria did some blocks of hydrotherapy, we asked for a copy of the program. This meant that Victoria could do some of the exercises at home in our pool, or any time we went as a family to the local pool. Or covertly, with occupational therapy we found that baking chocolate chip cookies from scratch, including rolling the mixture into all the little balls was an excellent activity involving both arms and hands.

Connect with other parents.

Today there are so many different ways to connect with parents who have children with similar needs. It is no longer just about chats in the therapist waiting room, resulting in new therapy ideas. There are many other methods of linking with other parents which means we are not isolated in caring for our disabled children. For example discussions via teleconference support groups; sharing ideas in an on-line forum and of course face to face support groups. So if you have a child with a disability, I strongly encourage you to seek out a connection strategy that suits your availability and personality. It is important as a carer not to become isolated.

I pray that these strategies will help you in your journey,

particularly if it is on-going like ours. As primary carers we need to ensure that we are looking after our health and well-being too, but more on self-care later in the book.

Chapter 5

More Therapy

EMAILS FROM 14TH MAR TO 18TH MAY 2011

EMAIL SENT ON 14TH MARCH 2011

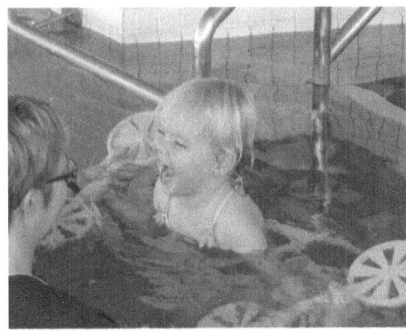

Victoria's first hydrotherapy session at Rankin Park, Newcastle

Firstly, thank you so much for your prayers. Victoria is continuing to make great steps forward with her left side motor skills. We started hydrotherapy last week, and what fun she had, as you can see by the photo. There was lots of walking, ball throwing and riding on noodles. We are scheduled to do this therapy once a week. It was good to see Victoria enjoying the water again.

Today we went to the Physio and OT at the hospital. The

therapist's feedback on Victoria's left arm, hand and fingers was very positive. The night hand splint has been making a big difference to her finger extension. So, as Victoria is so amenable to wearing the splint at night time, the therapists have now made an additional splint for her to wear from her wrist to the upper arm, to help keep the arm muscles lengthened out. We are so grateful for these therapist's diligence and care that they are taking with our precious daughter.

The feedback on Victoria's walking was not quite so positive today. For some reason, unknown at this stage, the limping has become more pronounced during the past week or so. I found this news very upsetting and my mind started to wander into her future, and what it would hold. The tears did flow this afternoon. I have been waiting for them to come for a while. When I spoke to Ken about this he reminded me that it is better to have Victoria Grace with a limp, rather than no Victoria Grace, and that she has the strength of character and lovable personality to cope with whatever her future holds. How right he is.

So we continue to take one day at a time, and cast our cares on our faithful God.

> *Cast your cares on the LORD and he will sustain you; He will never let the righteous be shaken.*
> *(Psalm 55:22 NIV)*

Thank you again for your love, support and prayers.

MORE THERAPY

EMAIL SENT ON 30TH MARCH 2011

Thank you for your continued prayer support for Victoria Grace. In the past week or so we have witnessed a few breakthroughs:

- ✓ Victoria can now put her nightie on by herself

- ✓ Victoria can swim the length of our pool with her floaty on, kicking both legs and using both arms

- ✓ Victoria is no longer waking up through the night, so we are all getting a better night's sleep

Victoria's use of her left arm and hand continues to improve each week. This is very good news. Lots of activities including doing puzzles, Tupperware ball exercises, finding small blocks in a container of rice, throwing bean bags into hoops etc, are definitely helping, and I think Victoria herself can feel the improvements, as it becomes easier and easier for her to do these activities with the left hand. She is using her left hand more voluntarily in play to assist the right hand. While this is good, the OT said this morning that we need to continue working towards getting the left hand to be as dexterous as possible, so please continue to pray for full recovery for the left hand and fingers.

Victoria's balance and leg strength has also continued to improve. The hydrotherapy will continue for another 4 weeks and then there is a specialist swimming teacher who happens to teach at our local pool, only five minutes from home, hooray, so we will enrol Victoria there. She continues to love the hydrotherapy sessions.

There has not been much improvement with Victoria's actual walking, so the physiotherapist suggested that a thermoplastic splint worn during the day would help to improve her gait. The splint will be made and fitted over the next few weeks. It will probably come up to the back of her mid-calf and will fit into her shoe. From a confidence point of view, thankfully it is coming into winter, so long pretty socks and trousers will make it less visible for the next six months at least.

One thing I have been concerned about is whether Victoria will be able to start at Prep next year as Marshall and Charlotte have done when they were four years old. Today I plucked up enough courage to ask the OT about this and she assured me that there should be no reason why Victoria could not start in 2012. That was such a relief for me to hear. Victoria is so keen to go to Prep, and has been asking about it constantly.

As you may be able to tell from my comment above, the last few weeks have been a struggle for me emotionally. A few weeks ago I said to God, 'I haven't cried much since those first few days of the diagnosis, and I feel like I should be crying more'. Then a week later I had a session with a counsellor who said I needed to 'give myself permission to grieve for the plans and dreams I had for Victoria' so I have given myself permission and guess what, the tears have now been flowing everywhere – the shopping centre, the bus-stop, swimming lessons, school – you name it, they have arrived.

We went to the local supermarket last week and there were some ladies sitting at a table fundraising for the Ronald McDonald House. I took one look at the table and burst into tears. The comfort that the Ronald McDonald family room provided to us at the hospital is indescribable. It was a place we could go and feel a bit normal, rather than being stuck in the hospital room constantly reminded of our circumstances. I spent a good ten minutes crying with the ladies at the fundraising table – they of course were very understanding.

Now I am reading a book called Good Grief [9] – and think that I am somewhere in Stage Two - We express emotion, and Stage Three - We feel depressed and very lonely. Hopefully I won't be in those stages for too much longer. They suggest there are ten stages. Of course my ever-present God continually encourages me to ….

> *Have I not commanded you? Be strong and courageous. Do not be terrified; do not be discouraged, for the LORD your God will be with you wherever you go.* (Joshua 1:9 NIV)

I pray this for Victoria too.

Enough of my self- indulgence – thank you again so much for the prayer support and practical support we have been receiving, and for the encouraging replies to these emails. It certainly helps me to make it through another day.

EMAIL SENT ON 14TH APRIL 2011

Thank you for your prayers and support. We continue to see progress with Victoria's arm movements and fingers. Last week Victoria was picking up a pencil in her left hand and scribbling with it.

One big praise point of the past fortnight is that the hydrotherapy teacher advised that Victoria now didn't need to go to a specialist swimming teacher, she could return to her mainstream swimming class at the same swimming centre that Marshall and Charlotte go to. This is excellent news. While Victoria has loved the hydrotherapy, it will be good to go back to doing something 'normal' with her. Victoria will start the new swimming class next Thursday. It is wonderful to have more tangible progress.

As it is school holidays Marshall and Charlotte came to the hospital with us on Monday for the OT appointment. We wanted them to get a bit more understanding of what Victoria has to re-learn and meet some of the wonderful people that are helping her along this journey. Victoria also had her leg measured for the day-time splint. It will take about three weeks to be made and will be made out of very thin flower-patterned plastic. Every day since Monday Victoria has been asking, 'when will my flower splint be ready?' We are continually amazed at her compliance regarding the splints she has to wear. There has not been one complaint from her about them.

Another praise point is the four hours respite support we are receiving from the Hunter Brain Injury Respite Options organisation. They have some lovely ladies that come and play with Victoria each Friday at home. It gives me a bit of a break and provides Victoria with some new playmates.

We are so grateful for the improvements in Victoria's gross and fine motor skills and continue to believe in faith that the MRI scan scheduled for May 5th will show either no change or a reduction in the size of the residual tumour.

EMAIL SENT ON 30TH APRIL 2011

Well the last couple of weeks have been full of interesting goings on .....

Victoria enjoyed her first swimming lesson back at Coughlans Swim Centre. I cried for the first ten minutes, tears of joy at seeing Victoria back doing something that was 'normal'. She did very well kicking both legs and paddling with both hands. It was a good reminder of the progress she has made in the past three months since the operation.

When Victoria is very tired, or if she wakes up during the night, she is currently very reluctant to accept help from anyone except me. The psychologist at the hospital told us this is very normal for a child who has been through what Victoria has been through, it is 'an attachment issue'. Nevertheless it has been quite tiring and wearing for us all. So now we have a chart on the fridge, an idea of the psychologist, called 'Let people help', and every time Victoria lets someone other than mummy help her, then she gets a sticker. When the chart is full, we will go shopping for a toy. So far, so good, she has four stickers on the chart.

Wednesday early evening Victoria was trying to do a poo and was quite distraught, her left leg started shaking, which it has done on a few previous occasions but I have been able to stop it by putting my hand on it. The doctor advised that this happens when the brain is having difficulty sending messages to the leg. However, this time I could not stop the tremors and her leg continued to shake for about forty-five minutes. This was very distressing for both Victoria and myself. Ken was on his way home, so as soon as he arrived he took Victoria to the hospital, where they stayed until 11.30pm and she was checked out by various doctors who finally decided to send her home. This was a reminder to me of just how intricate the human body is and that there is still a great deal of healing required.

This week will be a big week for Victoria and us all. On Monday Victoria will get her 'flower splint' to wear on her leg during the day. She is still very excited about that. And then on Thursday she has the MRI. We will get the results of the scan on the following Monday 9th. We are getting better at being patient. Mum and dad arrive tomorrow to give us some emotional and practical support over the next couple of weeks. I can't wait to see them. They have not been here since early Feb, so will no doubt notice a great difference in Victoria's ability.

We are also going to attempt to do some intensive constraint therapy at home, while we have the help of mum and dad here. This involves Victoria wearing Charlie, the puppet glove, on her right hand for two hours a day for two weeks. The two hours will be filled with specific activities using the left hand alone, accompanied by lots of praise and encouragement. The OT has advised that recent research has suggested that this type of intense therapy over a continuous period has proved very beneficial. We pray that this will be our experience.

So it has been an eventful couple of weeks, and it will be an eventful couple of weeks. Thank you again for your continued prayer support, the little victories each day remind us that God is in the midst.

EMAIL SENT ON 6TH MAY 2011

But he said to me 'My grace is sufficient for you, for my power is made perfect in weakness'
(2 Corinthians 12:9 NIV)

VICTORIA GRACE

God's grace is what we experienced yesterday as we waited to see Victoria after her MRI.

We knew that Thursday, yesterday, was about getting Victoria through the scan 'process' with minimal fuss and alarm, and thought that we would then have to wait until Monday to get the results.

As we sat waiting to see Victoria after the MRI, the Neurosurgeon who had operated on Victoria walked past and inquired why we were at the hospital. We explained and then Ken asked him if he could have a quick look at the scans now and let us know the results. There were only two people in the hospital who could do this for us, and one of them 'just happened' to walk by at the time we were sitting there.

He returned to tell us the great news that there had been no change in the residual tumour since the operation in January. Praise God.

Thank you again for your prayers and messages of support. We know we are blessed to have you on this journey with us. Love Ken, Wendy and family.

PS: After a bit of a mix up it turned out that the day leg splint was not ready last Monday, so we are hoping to get it this Monday. It was my turn to be gracious, with God's help of course.

MORE THERAPY

EMAIL SENT ON 18TH MAY 2011

Well, finally the day splint has arrived. As you can see by the photo it is as feminine as possible, with butterflies imprinted on the plastic.

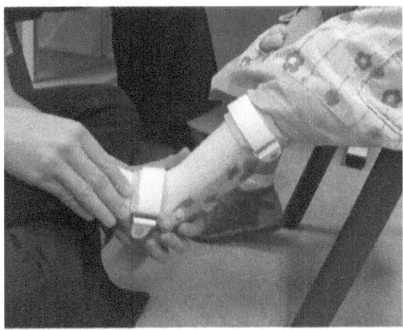

Victoria having her first splint (AFO – Ankle Foot Orthosis) fitted at the Physiotherapy Department at John Hunter Children's Hospital.

The physio suggested that Victoria might only wear it two hours in the morning and two hours in the afternoon for a week or so until she gets used to it. But in true Victoria style, this 'getting used to it period' has not been required; she wore it for eight hours yesterday, and still has it on today as I write this email.

Victoria's walking is a lot more stable with the splint on. The aim of the splint is to prevent her gait getting worse than it is now. We pray that this will be the case, and that in fact her walking will be improved when she does not wear the splint.

One small challenge with the splint is that, when Victoria has the splint on, she actually has two different size feet due to the sole on the splint – left foot – size eleven, right foot – size nine, so shoe shopping on Monday was fun. Praise God we had an excellent shop assistant helping us.

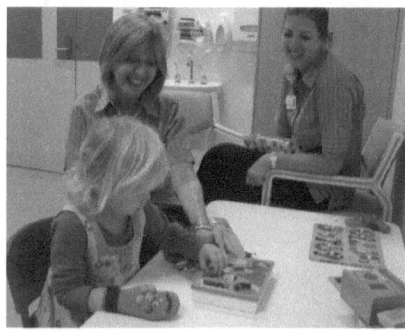

Victoria's therapy session wearing 'Charlie' at the Occupational Therapy Department at John Hunter Children's Hospital.

The other photo I have attached shows Victoria doing an occupational therapy session. Victoria is wearing 'Charlie' on her right hand, to ensure the left hand does all the work. The OT continues to be amazed at Victoria's progress with her hand and arm. Her physio is in the background.

During the review of the scan last week it was found that Victoria had suffered a small stroke during the operation. The Doctor has advised that this would mean the rehabilitation would take longer.

Thank you for continuing to pray for full recovery of Victoria's left side, and also that Victoria will not lose the wonderful confidence she has as she wears this splint in her everyday life.

MORE THERAPY

REFLECTION – CREATIVITY IN THERAPY

Initially, every time I went to Victoria's therapy appointments I was filled with trepidation. What little surprises were in store for us today? Would the report be favourable or otherwise? What new activity would we have to incorporate into our already full routine?

Over time I began to realise that hemiplegia is not a stable condition. Its effects can differ each day, month or year. You never know what the situation will be from appointment to appointment.

> *Don't expect doctors and therapists to be able to tell you how a child will progress, as each child's hemiplegia is different..... Hemiplegia also does not grow worse, but its effects may become more obvious as time goes on.... As children with hemiplegia grow, their muscles may become stiffer and they may need more treatment or even surgery.* [10]

For Victoria the amount of use her muscles get is definitely a factor that influences her muscle strength and range of movement. We stopped doing hand and arm exercises during one Christmas holiday period. We were caught up in enjoying the seven weeks of summer holidays and the festive season. In February we visited the OT for a review appointment. Sadly Victoria had lost a substantial amount of the hand and arm function she had worked so hard to gain over the previous twelve months.

I found this appointment confronting. The stark realisation hit me; this really was a use-it-or-lose-it situation. As a friend with medical knowledge in this area told me,

'The brain also has some plasticity in children so functions can move from a damaged area to another area.'

With Victoria being a young child, the responsibility fell to me, the primary care giver, to ensure that she used it. This responsibility weighed heavily on my heart and still does today. One of my biggest fears was that Victoria would become an adult with a withered left hand that was of no functional use to her. In the early days around our home you would often here the phrases, 'Please use your left hand' or 'Can your left hand help with that?'

The prevailing medical perspective on hemiplegia is,

> *Hemiplegia is what is called a chronic condition: it will not get better, but your child can be helped to get the best use out of the affected arm and leg, and will find all sorts of ways of getting around the practical challenges that life throws at them.* [11]

However, I firmly believe that our God can intervene and reverse the effects of hemiplegia. This may sound impossible to readers who don't share the same faith as me. I am a believer in Jesus Christ and his healing power.

MORE THERAPY

The Bible, in Isaiah 53, clearly says that Jesus bore all our diseases and infirmities when He died on the cross. I believe Jesus has provided the healing for hemiplegia too. There is an example of Jesus' healing power in the Gospel of Luke.

> *But He was aware all along of their thoughts, and He said to the man with the withered hand, Come and stand here in the midst. And he arose and stood there. Then Jesus said to them, I ask you, is it lawful and right on the Sabbath to do good [so that someone derives advantage from it] or to do evil, to save a life [and make a soul safe] or to destroy it? Then He glanced around at them all and said to the man, Stretch out your hand! And he did so, and his hand was fully restored like the other one.* (Luke 6:8-10)

While we are waiting to see the manifestation of Jesus' healing power in Victoria's body, we will continue with the therapy routines. We will carry on doing whatever we can to help her get the most use possible from her left arm and hand.

When Victoria was about seven years old, she realised that her left hand was smaller than her right hand, and started calling it, 'my little hand'. I would often hear her talking to her siblings, putting her two hands together and saying, 'look, my left hand is smaller than my right hand, isn't that cute.' There were a few occasions when she asked questions about the little hand, such as, 'Mummy, why is it smaller?' We had to explain that due to the stroke during her operation the messages from the brain weren't getting through to it properly. But, the more that she used it, the more it would grow and be a help to the rest of her body. And that we need to continue to pray for it to grow.

As Victoria gets older, she is starting to take more responsibility for managing the effects of hemiplegia. We work together to create activity plans that encourage full engagement of the left hand. Thankfully she has the capacity to understand, at an age appropriate level, the reasons for the exercises and the impacts of not doing them. Now six years on, the Occupational Therapist reports that she is still seeing gains in both strength and functionality, thanks to continuing regular therapy, and daily use of Victoria's left hand.

MORE THERAPY

In the previous chapter I said that it is challenging to keep a young child engaged in regular therapy, although with a very young child it is easy to make a game out of the therapy. Appendix C contains a list of the therapy activities, based on various sources, we found worked very well for younger children. Appendix D contains a sample of a one hour occupational therapy plan we often used at home.

My prayer is that this information will be useful to parents in similar situations.

Chapter 6

New Things and Events

EMAILS FROM 16TH JUN 2011 TO 30TH JAN 2012

EMAIL SENT ON 16TH JUNE 2011

Yesterday was a milestone day in Victoria's rehabilitation.

It was our last visit to the John Hunter Hospital for occupational therapy and physiotherapy. It was so sad to say good-bye to the lovely ladies who have so lovingly helped us tremendously since the beginning of this journey. And at the same time it was great to know that Victoria had reached the place of recovery where she could be transferred to the care of the community based Paediatric Brain Injury Rehabilitation Team (PBIRT). Praise God. Victoria's physical strength and ability continues to improve.

The care from the PBIRT team will begin with a number of assessments. Next week we will have a visit by the occupational therapist and social worker. The following week a neurological assessment will be done. Then in the next week a physiotherapy assessment will also be done. It was suggested by the oncology psychologist that speech therapy would also assist Victoria. The wonderful thing about the PBIRT is that all the help Victoria requires in these areas is available from the one team, so it is a co-ordinated integrated rehabilitation approach. We praise God for the wisdom and expertise within this team.

A couple of weeks ago I registered our family with the Camp Quality charity, whose slogan is 'Laughter is the best medicine'. They support families who have children with cancer, providing family fun days, family camps, childrens camps etc, all free. On Friday a package arrived from them, with t-shirts and hats for each child. Victoria and Alexandra wanted to wear theirs immediately.

In fact, the next day we were going to Sydney to visit some friends, and all the children wanted to wear them.

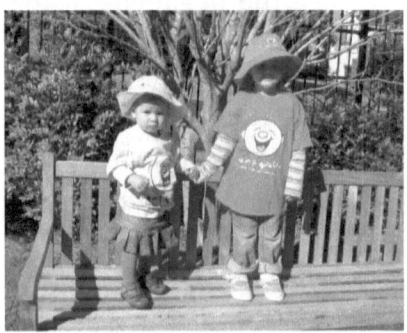

Alexandra and Victoria at home wearing their new Camp Quality T-shirts and Hats

We praise God for the people who set up these types of charities and the people who so faithfully donate time and money to them.

NEW THINGS AND EVENTS

The Camp Quality introduction was a clear reminder, that while there have been many negative things along this journey, there has also been so many positive, new things that our family has been able to experience. It has helped us all grow closer together, and get more of an understanding and empathy for families with children who suffer illness of any kind.

> *And we know that in all things God works for the good of those who love him, who have been called according to his purpose.* (Romans 8:28 NIV)

Thank you again for your prayers and support. We know that God is definitely in the midst and working in us, and hopefully through us.

EMAIL SENT ON 4TH AUGUST 2011

Victoria had another scan on Tuesday this week, we found out the results yesterday – the tumour continues to remain stable – awesome news!

Once again we praise God for His healing power, and for amazingly guiding the hands of neurosurgeon, which cut right into the centre of Victoria's brain appearing to cause virtually no additional damage. This has been confirmed by various cognitive assessments that have been completed on Victoria over the past month. The words of the paediatric neurologist regarding Victoria were 'she gives all the impressions of a very bright, alert, interested and intelligent child and I would be fairly optimistic.'

As you can see by the attached photo, taken a few weeks ago, Victoria is definitely back enjoying her life. The wonderful thing about this photo, is that 6 months ago, she could not lift her left arm or stretch out the fingers on her left hand – and now – well the photo shows it all.

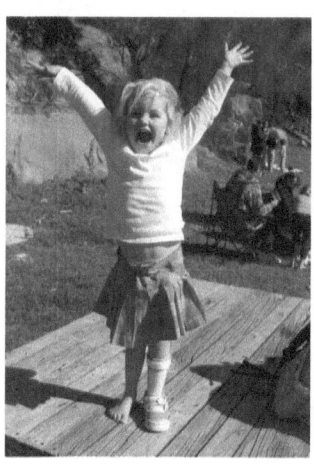

Victoria doing a star-jump at Brooklyn, NSW

Throughout this journey to date, God has provided us with the strength to get through each day and has continued to remind us that we need to do the following;

> *Let us then approach the throne of grace with confidence, so that we may receive mercy and find grace to help us in our time of need.* (Hebrews 4:16 NIV)

NEW THINGS AND EVENTS

Thank you again for your prayers and support.

EMAIL SENT ON 5TH SEPTEMBER 2011

Victoria has been progressing very well. In the last month we have received some good reports and made some excellent progress.

The Occupational Therapist and Physiotherapist carried out a Bayleys assessment on Victoria. The 'normal' range is from 8 to 12 (being the high end of 'normal'). Victoria's results were as follows – Cognitive = 12; Fine motor = 11; and get this, Gross motor = 8! So the prayer, therapy and exercises have definitely had a great impact. I cried when the therapist gave me these results.

The therapists also advised that it is probably no longer necessary for Victoria to wear the night boot and night arm splint – again a blessing. Even though Victoria never complained once in the 7 months of having to wear these aids at night, I am sure it mustn't have been very comfortable and they did take away her independence in relating to going to the toilet through the night.

We have just spent the weekend at a Camp Quality Family Camp at Myuna Bay Sport and Recreation Centre. We all had the best time. The children had a ball doing lots and lots of different activities – giant swing, flying fox, archery, rope walking, fishing and bike riding. And of course we met lots of wonderful people, both families who are doing the children with cancer journey and amazing volunteers whose aim was purely to ensure we were having fun. The photo I've attached shows Victoria doing the rope walking. In true Victoria style she was determined to give everything a go and where possible do it without assistance.

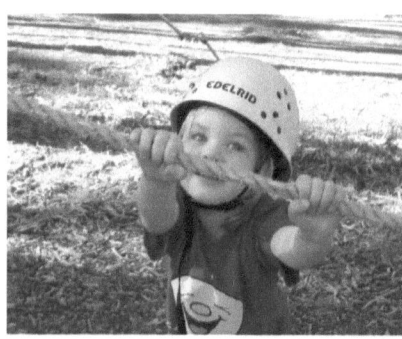

Victoria on the Low Ropes at the Camp Quality Family Camp.

We feel blessed to be witnessing such healing, and pray that the improvements will continue to come for Victoria. Thank you again for your prayers, love and support.

EMAIL SENT ON 3RD NOVEMBER 2011

Victoria had another MRI scan on Tuesday this week – actually scheduled for 3pm on Melbourne Cup day. Needless to say, the scan didn't happen until 4pm. We received the results yesterday, advising that the residual tumour continues to be stable. Praise God!

While we were looking at the scans on the light board with the neurosurgeon, Victoria was intrigued to see her round white eyeballs in one of the axial scans, and then commenced to draw a picture of her head and eyeballs. We are continually getting educated on this journey.

Victoria continues to progress well in all areas. She is now doing swimming lessons twice a week and can swim about 4 metres without any aids. I still cry when I watch her swimming, so determined to follow the teacher's directions and succeed.

Victoria is so excited about going to Prep next year, and while that may present her with some challenges physically, we are believing that with her determination, personality and God on her side, she will continue to succeed at all that she does.

Thank you so much for all the prayer and support for Victoria and our family in the past 10 months. Victoria is a living testimony to God's grace and faithfulness.

EMAIL SENT ON 30TH JANUARY 2012

Well, it is just over a year since Victoria had the operation to remove most of the brain tumour, and what a year it has been. A year of healing and going from strength to strength, all under the covering of God's amazing grace.

One week ago we met with the OT who did a school readiness assessment on Victoria, keeping in mind that after the operation twelve months ago Victoria could not lift anything with her left hand, as it had very little strength and mobility, even Twinkle Twinkle Little Star was impossible for her to do. Towards the end of the assessment the OT asked me if I was particularly concerned about anything, I replied, no not really. The OT then said to me that Victoria can do everything required for the school readiness assessment. Praise God

Her leg continues to strengthen; she can almost balance on the left leg now for one second. Botox treatment is being considered for blocking the muscle contractions (spasms). The administration of the Botox is done under a general anaesthetic by an orthopaedic surgeon. If it works, it is effective for three to six months, and then it would have to be administered regularly.

Last week we got a new splint, that should last twelve months. Buying school shoes was a little challenging, with difficulties finding a style the splint will fit into. Once again due to its extra length we had to buy two different sizes in the same shoe – Victoria found this quite amusing, wanting to know which shoe was the 'adult size' and which one the 'child size'. She was laughing and I was crying!

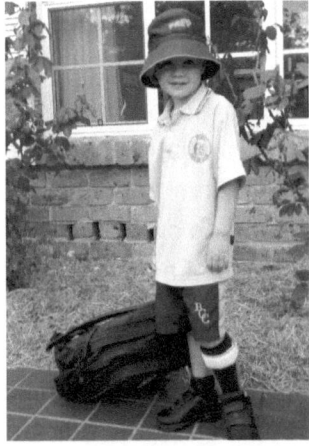

Victoria's first day at Prep at Belmont Christian College

As for today, saying good bye to her at Prep was another time for tears, for me, not Victoria. Twelve months ago we didn't know if this day would be possible, so to witness her today, in the prep classroom doing the various activities was a blessing beyond words.

Victoria's next scan is scheduled for February 9th, next week. We are believing that the results will continue to be stable.

Thank you again for your prayers and practical help during the past 12 months. Your love, support and encouragement has helped to get us to this remarkable day.

VICTORIA GRACE

REFLECTION – CAMP QUALITY MEETS OUR NEEDS

After Victoria was discharged from hospital, all her oncology appointments were in the Paediatric Oncology Day Unit. While sitting in the waiting room I would often read the notice boards. I always skimmed over the Camp Quality posters, thinking our family didn't need that sort of help. We are doing fine. How wrong I was.

Now, when I reflect on that time, I think that I was really in denial of what we had been through, how our life had changed, combined with a deep longing for how it used to be. I didn't want to 'need' an organisation like Camp Quality.

However, as you've read in this chapter, five months after Victoria's diagnosis, I had come to a place where I thought, "Yes, we do need this organisation. They are there for families like ours. We need some fun in our lives again", so I registered our family. When the initial introduction package of Camp Quality T-shirts and hats arrived, I just cried.

Many people had been so kind and generous to us over the past five months. But this was something different. We had never been on the receiving end of a charity organisation before. It is a very humbling experience, receiving gifts from people you don't know.

One of the best things about Camp Quality (CQ) is that

it doesn't only provide support for the child who has cancer, it provides support for the entire family, as its website says,

> Camp Quality's purpose is to create a better life for every child living with cancer in Australia. ... Right from diagnosis, throughout treatment and in remission or bereavement, our programs support the whole family; at hospital, at home, back at school and away from it all.
>
> This means we support the mums, dads and siblings of kids with cancer too; our research shows that cancer has a huge impact on them and they often feel neglected by support that focuses solely on the child with cancer. This makes our inclusion of these family members across our programs unique, essential and urgent – so they can quickly form a solid support network around their brother/sister or son/daughter with cancer. [12]

In September 2011 we went to the first of many Family Camps. These gave us an opportunity to get away and learn how to be a family again with our new 'normal'. Participating in activities like archery, mud runs, giant swings, or just having water fights, allowed us to laugh again together. They created new fun family memories, helping to push the hospital memories into the background. The camps provided an environment in which we could talk, if we wanted to, to other families who understood what it is like to be on this journey.

The Camp Quality volunteers at every camp have been outstanding. On our first camp, Ken was quite unwell and unable to assist much with the children. The volunteers were always looking for ways to help me with them. The children were aged one, three, five and seven, so a lot of help was required. The volunteers are extremely well trained, being alert and sensitive to physical needs and also to the families' emotional needs. Not once has a volunteer initiated a conversation about Victoria's health and well-being. They just do not go there unless we initiate the conversation, and even then they simply provide a quiet, trained listening ear.

The Family Camps are only one part of the CQ program. As you read through this book, you will read about many other ways CQ has helped our family, including the Primary School Education Program with their puppets, Child Life Therapists in the hospital, Family Fun Days, Mother/Daughter camps and Father/Son camps. We have also had many memorable family holidays at their cabin at One Mile Beach, Port Stephens.

Every aspect of these programs helps members of our family in different ways. The interaction with other parents in a relaxed atmosphere has been of great benefit to Ken and me. On more recent camps, the parents have gone out for a group dinner, while the children are supervised back at the camp. These have been fabulous nights out, providing a stress-free setting to chat about whatever we wanted, the cancer journey or other things happening in our lives.

Our children have grown in confidence as they've participated in various physical challenges. Charlotte took up the sport of Rock Climbing, after enjoying it so much at a camp. The children also have opportunities to go on camps without their parents. Charlotte and Victoria went on their first camp to Dubbo, NSW, five hours drive away, for four nights when they were aged only six and four. I think it was a little challenging for their companions, but our girls still laugh about various events that took place on that camp. Marshall had such a good time at the CQ camps, that when the time came to go on school camp he got a bit of shock. He had to keep his cabin tidy. This wasn't a requirement at CQ camps. Their camps are purely about the kids having fun.

But in that fun environment, there is that underlying goal of building resilience in children whose childhood has been cruelly interrupted by cancer. We are so grateful to this organisation and all it has given us.

I know that many of the people who donate time and money probably do not share the faith that we have, although I'm sure some do. However, it has not escaped me that they are all doing exactly what God asks us to do in Hebrews 10:24.

VICTORIA GRACE

And let us consider and give attentive, continuous care to watching over one another, studying how we may stir up (stimulate and incite) to love and helpful deeds and noble activities. (Hebrews 10:24)

Thank you to everyone who has ever given their money or time to Camp Quality. You have made a huge, tangible difference in the lives of many families, including ours.

Chapter 7

The News We Didn't Want

EMAILS FROM 22ND FEB TO 18TH JUN 2012

EMAIL SENT ON 22ND FEBRUARY 2012

As you know Victoria had another scan on 9th February 2012. The analysis of the scan indicates that the residual tumour has grown by 2mm.

The doctors will wait until the next scan in June before making a decision on what action to take, most likely surgery again.

We were not expecting this news. It is a shock. The tears have flowed and the cries have gone out to God. We know that our God has been so faithful in this journey to date, and we choose to believe that He will continue to be faithful.

> *As you know, we consider blessed those who have persevered. You have heard of Job's perseverance*

and have seen what the Lord finally brought about. The Lord is full of compassion and mercy. (James 5:11 NIV)

We will continue to seek God for healing for Victoria, wisdom for the doctors and joy and peace to reign in our family as we embark on the next stage of this journey. From now until the scan on June 12th, we will be fasting every Tuesday, so if you feel led to join in this fast, or give up some type of food or drink for the day, for healing, please do.

At this time our children are not aware of what changes have taken place, and we appreciate your sensitivity in not discussing this change in their presence.

But as always in the time of despair there can be found moments of joy. We just spent a wonderful weekend at Riverwood Downs, Barrington Tops with Camp Quality, and enjoyed many wonderful activities like river tubing and horse-riding. Ken rode a horse for the very first time. I went tubing down the river with Marshall and got caught on a few rocks. Victoria and Charlotte spent a lot of time in the craft room and also enjoyed the horse-riding.

For anyone who is interested to know more about fasting for spiritual purposes, Jentzen Franklin's excellent book Fasting, gives a very good explanation. Here is an excerpt from his book,

What is fasting? ... Stated simply, biblical fasting is refraining from food for a spiritual purpose... When you eliminate food from your diet for a number of days, your spirit becomes uncluttered by the things of this world and amazingly sensitive to the things of God... During the years that Jesus walked this earth, He devoted time to teaching His disciples the principles of the kingdom of God...

In the Beatitudes, specifically in Matthew 6, Jesus provided the pattern by which each of us is to live as a child of God. That pattern addressed three specific duties of a Christian: giving, praying, and fasting. Jesus said, "When you give ..." and "When you pray ..." and "When you fast." He made it clear that fasting, like giving and praying, was a normal part of Christian life. As much attention should be given to fasting as is given to giving and to praying. [13]

> *He talks about Jesus' example of fasting in the desert and his teaching about fasting in Matthew 17. Franklin asks these questions,*
>
> *If Jesus could have accomplished all He came to do without fasting, why would He fast? The Son of God fasted because He knew there were supernatural things that could only be released that way. How much more should fasting be a common practice in our lives?* [14]

EMAIL SENT ON 4TH MAY 2012

Well it has been another day charged with emotions.

Victoria's physio phoned us on Wednesday to say that a spot had become available in a ten week hippotherapy program, at the Riding for Disabled Centre at Raymond Terrace. This program is run once a year for four children only, and she was wondering if Victoria would be interested in going. What favour for our beautiful girl. Of course we accepted the invitation instantly.

I started to cry as soon as we drove in through the gate of the centre, knowing that these professionals, two physios, one OT and four other volunteers had given up their time today to provide this opportunity for Victoria and the three other children. Victoria absolutely loved the session, listening attentively and responding to all the instructions. It will be fascinating to see what developments take place over the next ten weeks.

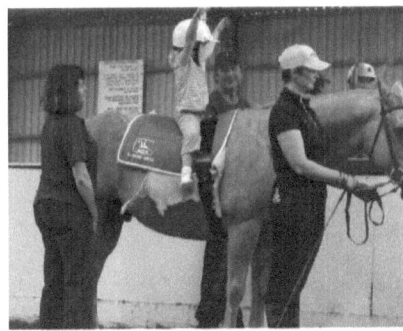

Victoria's first hippotherapy session on Wedge at the Riding for the Disabled centre.

Victoria's left side continues to strengthen with the daily activities at Prep, bike riding, swimming and some soccer coaching from Marshall. Her confidence with physical activities is increasing too. At Easter she swam off the boat without needing me to come in the water with her – another breakthrough.

These improvements are reflected in the physio appointments which are now only every three months and the OT appointments, which are every month. The progress Victoria has made is so wonderful to see, and we give glory to our faithful God.

The date of Victoria's next scan draws nearer, June 12. The closer it draws, the more it starts to consume our thoughts. It is sometimes a battle to take those thoughts captive and know that our God is in control. One of the scriptures that helps me daily is on the wall in front of my laptop as a good reminder that we cannot do this journey alone.

> *I look up to the mountain – does my help come from here? My help comes from the LORD, who made the heavens and earth!* (Psalm 121:1-2 NLT)

Thank you again for your prayers, support and encouragement.

EMAIL SENT ON 1ST JUNE 2012

Well, we have had some great news regarding Victoria since my last email. Thanks to all those people who have been praying and fasting.

As you may remember Victoria had a referral made earlier this year to have Botox injections in her left leg to help reduce the clonus (uncontrollable shaking of her left leg when she puts it in a particular position). In late April, Victoria's physio felt that the Botox would still be of benefit for her leg and was following up the referral (which was now at Westmead Children's hospital in Sydney, due to a re-structure up here).

We were given an appointment in Sydney for 23rd May,

and Victoria's physio wanted to do an assessment on her before the Sydney visit. During this assessment appointment in mid-May, the physio said that there had been such a big improvement with Victoria's walking in the past three weeks, that she felt the Botox would now not be of any benefit to Victoria. The Sydney appointment was cancelled. We praise God for this positive report, as we feel the less chemical intervention, the better.

The hippotherapy program with Wedge, the horse, continues to go well. We have two sessions left. Victoria loves it, and it has definitely contributed to the walking improvements we have seen. The hippotherapist has asked if Victoria would take part in a hippotherapy training session being conducted by a Canadian hippotherapist in late July, training fifteen Australian physios. Another great opportunity.

After each hippotherapy session the girls love to go exploring in the sensory garden next to the riding centre. It is filled with 'junk' that the children can touch, smell and play with. They absolutely love it.

On Monday this week, Victoria's Occupational Therapist suggested that we should undertake an eight week, two hours per day Constraint Induced Movement Therapy program at home. The purpose of this therapy is to improve the strength of Victoria's left hand, and also her left arm strength and stability. It involves the use of a glove on Victoria's left hand. Some of you may remember 'Charlie', from when we did similar therapy for five months after Victoria's operation. This time we have a green, water friendly glove and a floral glove. Within ten minutes of receiving the gloves, Victoria had named them, Ken and Alisa, and they are married.

Conducting this therapy is going to be a huge challenge for me, and I have been grateful to have my wonderful sister here this week to help me plan the program, and get the resources necessary. Secondly I am so grateful for the wonderful support network who responded to my request for help, as unlike last year when we did this therapy during the daytime, with Victoria at Prep three days a week, now this therapy has to be fitted in after school and needs my full attention. I need some extra hands around the home to help with Marshall, Charlotte and Alexandra. Thirdly, I am so grateful that through the generosity of some friends providing accommodation, my mum, dad and aunts will be visiting for four of the eight weeks. We thank God for his continued provision in our lives.

And of course we have the next scan on June 12th, and will not get the results until Monday 18th June. Thank you to all those people who are standing with us in prayer and fasting for a good result.

> *Fixing our eyes on Jesus, the pioneer and perfecter of our faith. For the joy set before him he endured the cross, scorning its shame, and sat down at*

the right hand of the throne of God. Consider him who endured such opposition from sinners, so that you will not grow weary and lose heart. (Hebrews 12:2-3 NIV)

Thank you once again for your support on this journey.

EMAIL SENT ON 13TH JUNE 2012

Thank you to everyone who was praying for us on Tuesday. We had an amazing day.

I took the four children to the hospital, sort of like an excursion, and a wonderful neighbour to help me out for the times when I needed to be with just Victoria. I really wanted Marshall and Charlotte to get a bit more of an understanding about what Victoria has to go through with the fasting, general anaesthetic and recovery, and just a general reminder about the hospital environment.

Well, I think they understood about the fasting. They were very considerate about not eating in front of Victoria. I know they definitely got a very good understanding of the Starlight Express room with all the Wii games, DS's, Play Stations and craft activities.

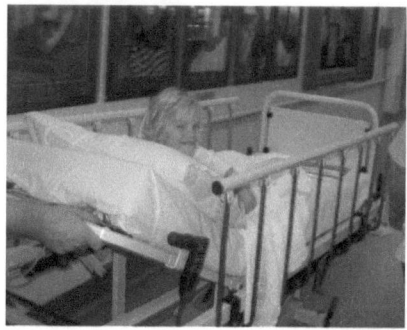

Victoria in the John Hunter Hospital's main corridor

Victoria herself thought it was wonderful having all her siblings with her, especially when it was time to go down for the MRI and we all went with her through the corridors. All the other people had to make way for us, and I saw quite a few smiles on people's faces as they realised that this was definitely a family affair.

Previously when it had been time for Victoria to have the gas for the anaesthetic, the anaesthetist would hold the mask over her mouth, but this time he asked Victoria to do it herself, which she did so very obligingly. We are so blessed to have a 4 year old who handles these events so maturely.

While we were at the hospital, we met with the OT for a review of the effectiveness of the constraint therapy. The OT was very impressed that Victoria was voluntarily using her left hand more, meaning less prompting required, and also that the strength in her left shoulder and arm had improved, after only one and a half weeks of the eight week program. To give you an example of the improvement, during the first few days Victoria could only lift a toy teapot quarter full of water with her left hand and arm. Now she can lift the toy teapot completely full of water. We praise God for this quick result, and look forward to the improvements that the next six and a half weeks will bring. And we thank God for our friends and family who have so generously given their time, enabling us to do this therapy program.

Thank you again for your prayers for Victoria and for our entire family. One scripture that has sustained me for the past week has been,

> *No test or temptation that comes your way is beyond the course of what others have had to face. All you need to remember is that God will never let you down; he'll never let you be pushed past your limit, He'll always be there to help you through it.*
> (1 Corinthians 10:13 The Message)

I know that will be the truth regardless of the results we receive on Monday.

EMAIL SENT ON 18TH JUNE 2012

This is just a very quick update on what we have learnt this morning. The oncologist has advised that the tumour has grown appreciably.

There are three options:

- Chemotherapy – would start in two to three weeks' time

- Radiation therapy – not likely

- Surgery – possible, but high risk

He will be discussing the options with the neurosurgeon this afternoon. We should have a plan of action by end of tomorrow. Please pray for wisdom in this decision making process. I will be in contact in the next couple of days as to the decision regarding the treatment.

THE NEWS WE DIDN'T WANT

REFLECTION – DEALING WITH DISAPPOINTMENT

Within eighteen months we had gone from receiving the devastating news that our daughter had a brain tumour requiring eight and a half hours of brain surgery; followed by six months of intensive physiotherapy, hydrotherapy, occupational therapy and hippotherapy.

Then we embarked on the emotional journey of accepting that we had a child with a physical disability and commenced building a new 'normal' life for our family. Now we were faced with the knowledge that the tumour had grown by 40% in four months. We were staring down the possible path of eighteen months of weekly chemotherapy treatment for our four year old daughter.

What do you do?

Where do you turn?

For me, there was only one thing to do. Pray. Call out to my God. He's the one I turn to. He is a safe place. I can tell Him I am angry, I am disappointed. He listens to me. He doesn't judge me. I love Him.

> *I love you, God – you make me strong. God is my bedrock under my feet, the castle in which I live, my rescuing knight. My God – the high crag when I run for dear life, hiding behind the boulders, safe in the granite hideout. I sing to GOD, the*

> *Praise-Lofty, and find myself safe and saved.*
> *(Psalm 18:1-3 The Message)*

Sometimes things happen and we don't understand why. While we are on this earth, we may never understand why. In her book One Thousand Gifts, Ann Voskamp recounts a conversation with her brother-in-law about the passing of his two sons at a very young age, both from the same medical condition.

> *"You know ..." John's voice breaks into my memory and his gaze lingers, then turns again toward the waving wheat field. "Well, even with our boys ... I don't know why that all happened." He shrugs again. "But do I have to? ... Who knows? I don't mention it often, but sometimes I think of that story in the Old Testament. Can't remember what book, but you know – when God gave King Hezekiah fifteen more years of life? Because he prayed for it? But if Hezekiah had died when God first intended, Manasseh would never have been born. And what does the Bible say about Manasseh? Something to the effect that Manasseh had led the Israelites to do even more evil than all the heathen nations around Israel. Think of all the evil that would have been avoided if Hezekiah had died earlier, before Manasseh was born. I am not saying anything, either way, about anything."*

> *He's watching that sea of green rolling in winds. Then it comes slow, in a low, quiet voice that I have to strain to hear.*
>
> *"Just that maybe ... maybe you don't want to change the story, because you don't know what a different ending holds."*
>
> *The words I choked out that dying, ending day, echo. Pierce. There's a reason I am not writing the story and God is. He knows how it all works out, where it all leads, what it all means. I don't.* [15]

This very powerful passage has stayed in my mind because it reminds me that God always knows best. When we don't understand a situation and want answers, we have to get to a place where we can trust God. We have to be able to live abundantly without the answers.

For me, it is about learning to have full confidence in God at all times. Learning to completely trust that God has a plan, and trust that it is a good plan. Learning to do exactly what Psalm 62:8 calls us to do.

> *Trust in, lean on, rely on, and have confidence in Him at all times, you people; pour out your hearts before Him. God is refuge for us (a fortress and a high tower). Selah [pause, and calmly think of that]!* (Psalm 62:8)

For the sake of our own mental health and the well-being of those around us, we have to come to a place of acceptance of our circumstances, no matter how angry and disappointed we are. I knew I had to accept what was happening to Victoria and make a decision to either move forward with God, learning how to trust and rely on Him more, or stay in an abyss of self-pity and go further down that destructive path.

I chose to move forward with God, to make Him my refuge and my rock. I chose to trust Him despite the circumstances, and expect that He would deliver an abundant life for Victoria, and indeed for every member of our family.

> *The thief comes only in order to steal and kill and destroy. I came that they may have and enjoy life, and have it in abundance (to the full, till it overflows).* (John 10:10)

Chapter 8

Chemotherapy

EMAILS FROM 19TH JUN TO 22ND JUL 2012

EMAIL SENT ON 19TH JUNE 2012

What to say???? The scan indicates that the tumour has grown by approximately 40%. Both the neurosurgeon and the oncologist agreed that action needs to be taken.

It has been decided that Victoria will have chemotherapy, initially weekly for 3 months commencing on Thursday 12th July. At the end of 3 months, a scan will be done to determine the effect of the chemotherapy and then decide what action to take next.

Next Thursday, 28th June, she will have an operation under general anaesthetic to have a portacath inserted in her chest, so then she won't need a drip put into her hand each week. She will lose her hair within 4 to 5 weeks of commencing the therapy.

I will be continuing to fast every Tuesday for the next 3 months so feel free to join in – it doesn't need to be food, it could be TV for the day.

Why fast you may ask? Isaiah 58 explains the nature of true fasting. A friend encouraged us today that verse 8 and 9 are what we need to claim for Victoria:

> *Then your light will break forth like the dawn, and your healing will quickly appear; then your righteousness will go before you, and the glory of the LORD will be your rear guard. Then you will call, and the LORD will answer; you will cry for help, and he will say: Here am I.* (Isaiah 58:8-9 NIV)

Again, for those who are in our everyday life, we so appreciate your support and would ask that you please continue to be sensitive to our family, especially the children, and refrain from talking about this circumstance in front of them. We will be telling the children at the weekend about the chemotherapy treatment.

Thank you again for your love, prayers and help. We so need it in abundance.

EMAIL SENT ON 29TH JUNE 2012

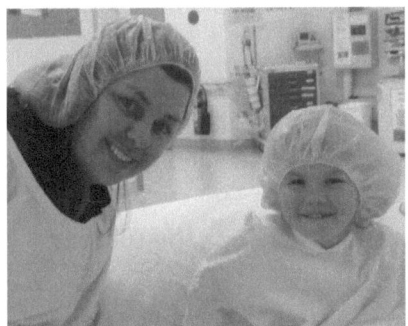

Victoria and I prior to Victoria having surgery for a portacath insertion at John Hunter Hospital.

Thank you for all the prayers that were said for us yesterday. Victoria's port insertion operation went very well. The surgeon was pleased with the ease with which the port and line went in, praise God.

Victoria was very grumpy when she woke up in the recovery room, in fact she screamed so loudly for so long, that the recovery staff didn't wait for the ward nurse to come and take us back to the ward, instead, the recovery nurses returned us to the ward themselves! Once we got back to the ward, Victoria promptly fell asleep for two hours, and then woke up to be her beautiful self again.

Here are a few of our prayer needs over the next three months

- ♥ Victoria will continue to know that she is loved by a faithful God and that she has what it takes to do this journey

- ♥ Wisdom and strength for Ken and I to continue to seek God's best for our family on this journey.

- ♥ No infection from the port

- ♥ No clots in the line connected to the port

- ♥ Chemotherapy treatment to shrink the tumour

- ♥ No side effects from the chemotherapy

Thank you again for your support and prayers. I know that our God is faithful and has perfect timing, although we don't always understand His ways. As we were waiting for Victoria to go in for the operation yesterday, God reminded me of the night before Victoria's brain surgery, when she started to vomit. The vomiting was an indication that the tumour was starting to have more serious impacts on her brain. He then reminded me how He brought her through that operation so wonderfully. This gave me a quiet confidence that He will do it again.

CHEMOTHERAPY

EMAIL SENT ON 13TH JULY 2012

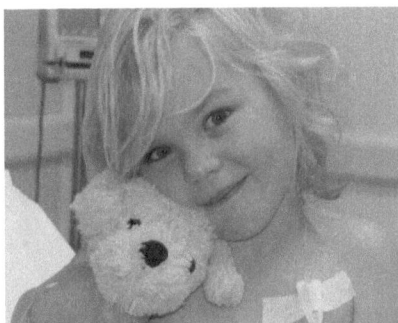

Victoria getting ready to receive chemotherapy treatment at John Hunter Children's Hospital

Well, we have started the next part of the journey, and what a start it was! Thank you for your prayers. It was clear to me at the hospital yesterday that once again God had gone before us and prepared the way.

The hospital staff were amazing, so aware of what is required to help the children in the best way possible. When it was Victoria's turn to commence treatment, the play therapist, Veronica, arrived and talked Victoria step by step through the process of accessing her port, and delivering the chemotherapy. She used teddy as the patient and Victoria took on the role of nurse.

This thoughtful preparation meant that when it was time for Victoria's port to be accessed, she didn't even wince, which is a huge blessing. As the nurse explained, if the first access is traumatic for the child, then subsequent accessing, in our case weekly for initially three months, maybe twelve months, continues to be traumatic. We thank God for His graciousness.

We were in the treatment room for about four hours. The actual chemotherapy infusion took only one hour and fifteen minutes. Victoria received the infusion through a tube under her shirt, directly into the port. Victoria was able to continue in her new role as 'nurse', bandaging teddy and Granny Bett's hand, eating and drinking or watching a DVD as she felt so inclined.

We returned home with a myriad of drugs and instructions including anti-nausea drugs, drugs to help prevent pneumonia and a mouth wash regime to be done four times a day to prevent mouth ulcers, which could be a bit challenging for a four year old. And so the journey continues.

Sometimes people ask me, How do you sleep at night? Aside from being 'pleasantly tired' most nights, just before I go to sleep, I roll over and read this scripture on the wall,

> *You will not have to fight this battle. Take up your positions; stand firm and see the deliverance the LORD will give you, O Judah and Jerusalem. Do not be afraid; do not be discouraged. Go out to face them tomorrow, and the LORD will be with you.*
> (2 Chronicles 20:17 NIV)

Thank you once again for the overwhelming support we continue to receive, not only the much needed and appreciated practical support, but all the emails and texts are so encouraging to us. And of course, thank you for petitioning heaven on Victoria's behalf.

EMAIL SENT ON 22ND JULY 2012

This is just a quick update to let you know that Victoria went through her 2nd round of chemotherapy with the same style as the first. She was very excited to go to hospital again and has accepted that this is now part of her weekly routine. Once again she experienced no nausea after the infusion, for which we are very grateful.

The magnitude of what we are dealing with was brought home to me yet again up at the hospital on Thursday, when I casually mentioned to the nurse that Victoria had started to wet the bed so I had put her in children's nappies to help both her and us get a good night's sleep.

'Oh' said the nurse, 'we must get you some purple elbow length gloves to put on while handling the used pullups, and some purple rubbish bags marked 'cytotoxic waste – incinerate' and you must bring them back to the hospital for us to dispose of. No-one is to touch her bodily fluids, especially in the first 48 hours after receiving treatment.'

Yet another bit of information to come to terms with.

Thank you again to everyone who is praying and providing us with practical support. You are testimony of God's continued provision in our lives, again, for which we are very thankful. My scripture for the day,

> *Rejoice in the Lord always. I will say it again: Rejoice!* (Philippians 4:4 NIV)

CHEMOTHERAPY

REFLECTION – THE CARER NEEDS TO BE CARED FOR

This reflection has been adapted from some blog posts I wrote for the ABC 'Speak Your Mind' project in late 2014.

Chronic illness takes a toll. Not only on the sufferer, but also on those who are caring for the sufferer and the siblings too. The emotional anguish and physical demands can be immense.

When Victoria was diagnosed with a brain tumour, we lived in survival mode for about six months. Then we experienced another major family trauma, Ken had a nervous breakdown, which led to a couple of weeks living in crisis mode and then a further six months in survival mode. 2011 was virtually a whole year wiped out.

Looking back, I can see that in February 2012, when the routine MRI indicated that the brain tumour was growing again, I experienced low level depression. Getting out of bed in the morning wasn't a problem. However there were periods of up to three months at a time, when I had trouble concentrating and was unable to clearly put thoughts together in my head. Often I experienced feelings of hopelessness. Thoughts that crept into my mind about the uncertainty of Victoria's future meant that some days I couldn't see the point in helping her keep up with her school work. I thought 'why bother if she isn't going to be here in a few years' time?' One night

I even dreamt about her funeral, the photos that would be displayed and the words we would share.

FIVE KEY STRATEGIES THAT HELPED WHEN I EXPERIENCED DEPRESSION

During these times of depression, there were five key strategies I used, by the grace of God, to help keep myself functioning.

Meditating on God's Word

I spent time daily regularly reading and re-reading scriptures that provided hope and reminded me that I was not alone in this darkness. I have mentioned these two scriptures previously. They were pivotal in helping me keep my focus on God.

> *You will not have to fight this battle. Take up your positions; stand firm and see the deliverance the LORD will give you, O Judah and Jerusalem. Do not be afraid; do not be discouraged. Go out to face them tomorrow, and the LORD will be with you.* (2 Chronicles 20:17 NIV)

> *Rejoice in the Lord always. I will say it again: Rejoice! Let your gentleness be evident to all. The Lord is near. Do not be anxious about anything, but in everything, by prayer and petition, with thanksgiving, present your*

requests to God. And the peace of God, which transcends all understanding, will guard your hearts and your minds in Christ Jesus. (Philippians 4:4-7 NIV)

Finding things to be grateful for despite the circumstances

Each morning when I wrote in my prayer journal I would start by finding something to be thankful for. Sometimes it was as simple, or as huge as 'Thank you God for helping me make it through yesterday'. I found that once I had made a start, it didn't take long to find more and more things to be thankful for.

Openly sharing my tears and fears with friends

Occasionally I knew I needed to have a good cry. I would go to a friend's house and knock on their door. When they opened the door, I just stood there and cried my heart out. They were so gracious to me, lovingly allowing me to grieve and express myself as and when I needed to.

Allowing my emotional state to be regularly monitored by my GP

In early 2012, after we had received the news that the tumour was growing again, I was at a regular check up with my GP. She saw I was struggling and suggested we meet every six weeks so she could assess my emotional state and determine if I needed any medication to manage the low level depression. Having this regular monitoring, knowing that someone else was reviewing how I was travelling emotionally gave me great comfort.

Asking for help

At this time our children were aged two, four, six and eight. They had many needs, both practical and emotional. I realised I was struggling to meet all their practical needs. There was absolutely zero capacity in me to even consider their emotional needs. Many days I recall thinking, if I just get the washing hung out today, it will be a good day. I knew I had to ask for help, something that wasn't easy for me to do, as I prided myself in being so independent and capable. However I realised if I didn't ask for help, our family's well-being was at risk. So I humbled myself and asked for assistance. It was one of the best strategies I employed as it reduced my responsibilities for a while giving me some much needed physical and mental rest.

FIVE KEY STRATEGIES FOR MAINTAINING MY MENTAL HEALTH

After eighteen months, around the time Victoria almost finished chemotherapy treatment, I began to move out of the mire of low level depression. My capacity to cope with life gradually increased. As I felt myself more able to deal with everyday life, I made the decision to equip myself with strategies to help me better manage my mental health in the future – prevention measures. I didn't have my head in the sand. I knew that while we continued to trust that God would heal our daughter, right now we had a child with a chronic illness and potentially many challenges ahead.

Here are the five main strategies I used to equip myself for on-going management of my mental health.

Understanding more about God's perspective on handling life's struggles

As a Christian who had relied so much on God to get me through the difficult times, I found myself wanting to understand more about His plan and purpose for our lives. In particular the way that the trials and tests we face refine our character and increase our faith. As it says in Romans,

> *Moreover [let us also be full of joy now!] let us exult and triumph in our troubles and rejoice in our sufferings, knowing that pressure and affliction and hardship produce patient and unswerving endurance. And endurance (fortitude) develops maturity of character (approved faith and tried integrity). And character [of this sort] produces [the habit of] joyful and confident hope of eternal salvation.* (Romans 5:3-4)

So I started increasing my daily devotional time with

God, including a combination of sitting in silence just waiting for Him to speak to me; worshipping; reading my Bible and reading various Christian devotion books. I was interested to find out how other Christians had coped with trials and their books seemed a logical place to start. Books like Something More [16] by Catherine Marshall, and One Thousand Gifts [17] by Ann Voskamp. When reading these books I found I could easily relate to the emotions these women experienced in times of trial, and also how their faith in God grew during these circumstances.

Seeking out information about caring for myself – the carer

I actively sought information about being a carer for someone with a chronic illness, which led me to various organisations, including one that ran a course for carers called 'Learning how to get better at caring for yourself'. It was a big effort to arrange child care so I could get to this course, however it was worth it. Taking the time to map out the areas of my life, my coping mechanisms, supports I had in place and then identify the gaps that needed to be filled, gave me a road map to move forward with.

Attending therapy and group counselling sessions

Due to the nature of our daughter's illness the hospital provided a psychologist experienced in paediatric oncology, to help patients, parents and siblings. For eight months I had monthly appointments with her to talk about all things related to our child's illness, especially the impact on our family and how I was, or was not coping. Again, knowing there were regular appointments scheduled helped me to feel less anxious about how I was travelling emotionally. I knew I had a professionally trained person keeping an eye on me. A few months after Victoria finished treatment, I was ready to share my thoughts and fears with a small group who had faced similar challenges. So I joined a tele-counselling group facilitated by Redkite, an Australian cancer charity that supports children and young people from 0 to 24 years with cancer and their families. The group focussed on transitioning from having a child receiving chemotherapy treatment to a 'new normal' life. It was fantastic to have the opportunity to share my thoughts and feelings in this environment, having people on the end of the phone say 'Yes I felt that too' or 'Yes I understand' knowing that they really did understand. Some of the group sessions were exhausting from re-living the various traumatic events. But overall the experience was very positive. It gave me a lot of clarity and positive reinforcement as it constantly highlighted how resilient we were despite the times when we had struggled emotionally.

Taking time out for myself

Further on in this book, I share about a day at the hospital, when I was a complete mess. I was crying and unable to have a coherent conversation with anyone. Another Mum looked at me, and gently said 'I have been where you are, you need to get away for at least 24 hours'. So with the help of family and friends, that is exactly what I did. I went away by myself, only 30 minutes from home, so I was nearby just in case there was an emergency. Nonetheless I was by myself, having respite for me. It was magnificent. In fact, it was so magnificent I made sure I had another time away booked in within the next three months. The break away from responsibilities and noise, enabled me to return to my family completely refreshed and ready to face the next challenge. Recognising I couldn't 'run away' for 24 hours every week, I started looking for a weekly activity that would enable me to 'escape' for an hour or so. I'd always had a passion for art, so I decided to enrol in drawing lessons. The lessons weren't in a formal classroom environment, rather they were in an artists' studio. There was full freedom to express myself through drawing within minimal structure. It was a creative therapy to help me process and in some ways escape from the trauma in our lives. What a blessing.

Choosing to eat healthier and exercise more

I had found the hospital environment extremely unconducive to looking after myself physically, both on the food (i.e. cafeteria food) and the exercise front. So as my mental health improved and we received an end-date for Victoria's chemotherapy treatment, I felt it was a good time to start improving my eating habits and regularly exercising. My improved healthy eating strategy involved introducing more raw fresh vegetables and reducing processed foods. For a period I followed the Fast Diet involving five days eating normally and two non-consecutive days eating up to 500 calories. This diet worked well with my very unpredictable life. There is anecdotal evidence that fasting has a positive impact on mental health. Exercising started with regular bike rides with a friend. My goal was to participate in a local annual fundraising bike ride, for the John Hunter Children's Hospital. The whole family was able to join in the bike ride at various stages which made for more great family memories. My exercise program gradually diversified to including weekly sessions at a local gym. These lifestyle changes have certainly helped to improve my physical and emotional stamina.

As a Carer, it is so important that we give priority to looking after our own spiritual, emotional and physical well-being.

> *Looking after parents' and carers' mental and physical health is just as important as looking after children's. When parents and carers look after themselves and feel supported, they are more able to provide their children with the best care they can. Having healthy parents and carers is also good for children's mental health and wellbeing. When parents and carers are more relaxed and less stressed, they are more able to relate to their children, make good decisions and model appropriate responses.* [18]

VICTORIA GRACE

Aside from the benefit to our own selves, it is in the best interests of those we are caring for that we are well – in every sense of the word.

Chapter 9

Wonderful Support

EMAILS FROM 1ST AUG TO 14TH SEP 2012

EMAIL SENT ON 1 AUGUST 2012

Thank you so much for the prayers for Victoria and our family. We witnessed God's perfect timing once again this week.

We had made a decision not to tell Victoria that her hair was likely to fall out as a result of the chemotherapy, until it actually started to fall out.

On Monday morning this week, I was combing her hair, and some hair did start to come out. That morning the Camp Quality puppets were scheduled to come to Prep to talk to the children about the physical effects of chemotherapy, specifically hair loss. So I decided not to say anything about the hair loss until after the Puppets had done their presentation.

The Camp Quality puppets were amazing, leaving the children with a couple of key messages – "you can't catch cancer", and "even though someone looks different now on the outside, they are the same on the inside". I sat at the back of the room, quietly crying throughout the presentation, finding it hard to believe that I was watching this show purposed that day for our daughter. We are just so grateful to these organisations that are established to help and educate in so many different ways.

Monday evening around the dinner table, we chatted about the puppets. I asked Victoria what she learnt about chemotherapy, and she said 'it makes your hair fall out', and I said, 'yes and that is probably what will happen to you, just like the puppet'. And then Victoria replied, 'It will grow back when I stop having the chemotherapy,' and I said 'yes'. And that was all there was to it. Since that conversation, she had shared this 'news' with a few people without any hint of anxiety or concern, for this response we give God the glory.

Thank you again for the wonderful support we have been receiving. Tiredness is a challenge for us all at this point in time, so we would very much appreciate prayer for supernatural strength, thanks. Isaiah 40:31 is a scripture we are standing on ...

> *But those who hope in the LORD will renew their strength. They will soar on wings like eagles; they will run and not grow weary, they will walk and not be faint.* (Isaiah 40:31 NIV)

EMAIL SENT ON 11 AUGUST 2012

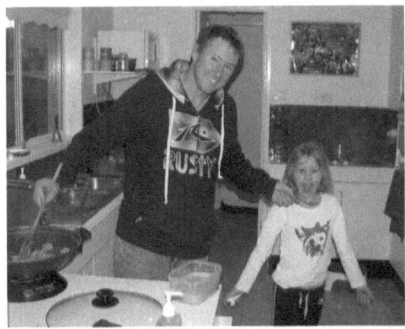

A family friend making dinner with Charlotte at our home

Today I would like to say a big 'Thank you' to everyone who has supported us along this journey, especially during these past few months since we learnt of this new stage we are in now. To be surrounded by such wonderful family and friends is truly amazing. Please indulge me as I share just a few examples of how we have been 'loved on.'

Family Support

My Mum, Dad and Sister came over from NZ in July to look after our four children, so Ken and I could have five nights away at Hillsong conference in Sydney, our first time away for that length of time by ourselves for nine years. And what a special time it was, sitting in the presence of God, feeding on His Word, getting rest and gathering strength for the journey ahead. Ken's Mum and Dad have been faithfully looking after Alexandra each Thursday since the chemotherapy started, as the treatment room is not really built for a two and half year old, again such a blessing for us. An extra blessing is to then come home to find that the kitchen floor has been washed and the ironing is all done.

School

Belmont Christian College, where Marshall, Charlotte and Victoria attend school, has just been fantastic with the support they have given our family. Nothing but love has been poured out on us. Victoria came home from Prep so excited this week because Prep had given her 3 beanies, and she excitedly announced that Prep was going to have a 'Beanie Day'. The staff at the hospital that visited the school to talk about Victoria, tell me each Thursday what a wonderful school it is, and that not all schools are so supportive. Once again, this is an example of God putting things in place long before we need them, as before we moved to Newcastle in 2006, God had told me that Belmont Christian College was where our children were to go to school.

Church

Macquarie Life Church, continues to provide prayer and practical support to our family. One of the pastors arrived with a trailer load of wood that he had cut himself for us. Almost every Sunday, someone from church gives us a meal to take home. Last week, some friends told me that they would love to come and clean our house. I graciously and very quickly accepted. We know we are part of such an exceptional huge God-centred family.

Friends

Thursdays are emotionally draining for me, when we return from hospital I run on automatic pilot until about five O'clock when I then start to emerge slowly out of a daze, knowing that there are four children that need dinner, homework time, and bedtime routine. One of my amazing friends has put together a dinner roster for Thursday nights for our family. A 'surprise' person calls me during the day to find out what time to deliver the meal. This is such a special moment in the day, another reminder that we are not on this journey alone. This week one friend arrived with wok in one hand and chicken and rice in the other, took over the kitchen and cooked a fantastic meal, ably assisted by Charlotte. I know there are many people who receive this email who don't live nearby, and I thank you for your emails and letters of support, encouragement and prayers. All are so necessary to get us through the more difficult days.

Support organisations for Children with Cancer

Camp Quality supports families of children with cancer so well. They think of every need. We have enjoyed their hospitality at Family Camps, a Mother and Daughter Camp, Sibling Camp, Dads and Lads Camp, family days and weeks away at their One Mile Beach cabin. These 'breaks' from life certainly help to revive us. My sister, on seeing the wonderful support Camp Quality has provided to us, has been donating her time and expert market research skills to Camp Quality New Zealand, designing and conducting national surveys of Camp Quality volunteers and families. A close friend here is having a fundraising event for Camp Quality. These are another two great flow-on effects of this circumstance. Redkite is another organisation that has been a wonderful help, providing financial assistance, particularly when Ken was unwell last year, and family fun days at Taronga Park Zoo and Ten Pin Bowling. Victoria also "qualifies" for a wish with the Starlight Children's Foundation, something special that we will look at doing in the next six months.

This journey may not be a short one. Depending on the outcome of Victoria's October MRI, we are possibly looking at twelve or more months of weekly chemotherapy sessions. So we are now moving into a phase of yet another new 'normal' for our family. In relation to the unfolding length of this journey, we do so appreciate the gifts that have been given to Victoria and know that they have come with much love, but in an effort to keep things 'normal' for our family, especially in relation to Marshall, Charlotte and Alexandra, we request that if you would like to give something, please consider making a donation to one of the amazing organisations that support families with children with Cancer, such as Camp Quality, Redkite, Ronald McDonald House or the Starlight Children's Foundation.

Thank you again for the love and support you have given our family, every single bit of it helps us to get through each week. Be encouraged:

> *You did not choose me, but I chose you and appointed you to go and bear fruit – fruit that will last. Then the Father will give you whatever you ask in my name. This is my command: Love each other.* (John 15:16 -17 NIV)

EMAIL SENT ON 23RD AUGUST 2012

What a wonderful week we have had at the Camp Quality Cabin at One Mile Beach, enjoying the beach and bike-riding, forgetting about the cares of this life. It has been a special week for all of us. We praise God that Victoria is well enough to join in all the family frivolity.

A month ago when we went bike riding as a family, Victoria did not appear to have the strength to push the peddles on her bike. For both Ken and me, this was distressing to watch.

So last week we took Victoria's bike with us on holiday in the hope that she could build up some strength and ride by herself. Well, every day she peddled her heart out, even after a big spill featuring quite a bit of blood. She desperately wanted to keep up with Marshall and Charlotte. This new found strength was great for Ken and me to see.

But what was even more heart-warming was to watch Victoria run in the front garden at home yesterday, without her splint on. She was pretty much running like a normal child. In fact if you didn't know her medical history, you wouldn't have noticed anything different in her running. This development was confirmed by her physiotherapist today. We thank God for the healing that is taking place, for whatever reason – riding the bike? Shrinking of the tumour? We don't know why, but we do know there has been a change.

> *But by the grace of God I am what I am, and His grace to me was not without effect. No, I worked harder than all of them – yet not I, but the grace of God that was with me.*
> (1 Corinthians 15:10 NIV)

We do have a couple of prayer points relating to the side effects of the chemotherapy treatment.

At the hospital today, Victoria was unable to have the chemotherapy treatment due to a low neutrophil count, less than 0.5, so we would appreciate your prayers for protection during this time of low immunity. Thank you.

For the past two months, Victoria has been losing weight. We have some strategies from the dietician at the hospital to help add extra calories to the small amounts of food she is able to eat, to increase her weight. So again, we would appreciate your prayers in this area.

WONDERFUL SUPPORT

Many thanks again for your prayer and practical support. It means so much to our family.

EMAIL SENT ON 1ST SEPTEMBER 2012

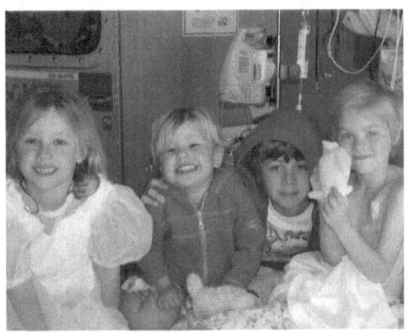

Charlotte, Alexandra, Marshall and Victoria in John Hunter Children's Hospital, J1 ward

Well, we are here in J1 Ward at the John Hunter Hospital. Ken brought Victoria up here last night after she was having some high temperatures and was generally looking unwell. Her neutrophil count on Thursday was lower than the previous week, 0.2.

As soon as Ken left home I texted a few friends asking for prayer for Victoria. Friday midnight when I spoke to Ken and the doctor, the doctor said her neutrophil count was now 1.1 and he didn't understand it.

Victoria's count had gone from 0.2 on Thursday to 1.1 by Friday night. This is not normal. Once I heard this news I was able to sleep peacefully for the rest of the night, knowing that God was truly in control. Unfortunately the same cannot be said for Ken, who had a night of not much sleep due to hospital responsibilities. Not the best way to start the celebration of his birthday today. The pancake breakfast has been postponed.

So it was good news on the count front, but Victoria has still been having high temperatures throughout the day. She will be in hospital until at least Monday morning, when the blood culture results will be returned, hopefully ruling out a bacterial infection.

My verse for the day,

> *Let us hold unswervingly to the hope we profess, for he who promised is faithful.* (Hebrews 10:23 NIV)

Thank you for your continued prayer and support.

EMAIL SENT ON 3RD SEPTEMBER 2012

Thank you everyone for your prayers over the past few days, and thank you to those who helped us out logistically with looking after children.

We thank God that Victoria could come home today, and give thanks we live in a place with wonderful medical expertise and support.

WONDERFUL SUPPORT

EMAIL SENT ON 14TH SEPTEMBER 2012

Thank you for your prayers, we have certainly needed them as these past two weeks have been very difficult for us all physically and emotionally. Some members of the family are still feeling the emotional effects of having Victoria in hospital for three days, and my being away from home to help her. Others have had a gastro bug, including myself, which has utterly drained us. Aquim gel has made a fortune from us as we have bottles in almost every room of the house, in an effort to stop the spread of the bug, especially to Victoria.

Hopefully now we are coming to the end of this time, with full health returning to all of us, and school holidays not far away to provide some much needed time for emotional healing and bonding within our family.

Of course during this time there have been some moments of joy. On the Sunday when Victoria was in hospital, a pet therapist came in with her dog. Victoria was well enough to pat the dog and feed him. This is just another wonderful example of people giving up their time to help children in need.

And then there was last night, the school musical, held at the Civic Theatre in Newcastle, where the Prep children got to do a 10 minute pre-show performance. From the moment they stepped on stage I cried. For there was Victoria, who only six hours earlier was sitting in hospital having the weekly chemotherapy, and now up on the stage, dancing her heart out in her fairy costume and having an absolute ball. She was living her life to the full and nothing was going to stop her.

Treatment-wise, next Thursday will be the last of this chemotherapy 'program'. Victoria will have a two week break, and then the Oncologist's plan is that she will commence another three months of weekly treatments on October 11th. This plan could change depending on the results of the MRI scheduled 9th October. Again we wait and with faith believe our God is in control.

> *Because of the LORD's great love we are not consumed, for his compassions never fail. They are new every morning; great is your faithfulness. I say to myself, 'The LORD is my portion; therefore I will wait for him.'* (Lamentations 3:22 -24 NIV)

Thank you again for standing with us in prayer and fasting, and for all the hands-on support.

REFLECTION – COMMUNITY, GIVING AND RECEIVING

We are so grateful for all the people who have stood with us in prayer and have supported us in so many different ways during these years. It has been, and still is, community in action. Community as God designed it to be, people loving each other through extremely difficult and testing times. People coming together and lifting the arms of the weary when the going gets tough.

> *This is My commandment: that you love one another [just] as I have loved you.* (John 15:12)

There is a temptation in the challenging times to become isolated, not wanting to connect with the world outside. Particularly when other people's lives seem so perfect, compared to your world which is quickly falling apart. We are not designed to live alone, especially not in the difficult seasons of life. It is humbling to reach out and ask for help, to admit that we cannot cope, to admit that we need others, especially God.

Community doesn't just happen. We need to be intentional about creating or being part of a community. This means reaching out to others, allowing yourself to be vulnerable in being first to offer the hand of friendship. One of our neighbours demonstrated this so well. On the day we moved into our home at Lake Macquarie, there was a note in our letter box. It contained key information about the area, including the phone number of the local fish and chip shop. She had left some milk and bread for us at our front door. That thoughtful act has led to over ten years of lovely friendship.

Following that act of kindness, our family decided to host a Christmas party for our neighbours. It was a party full of fun, providing an environment for many neighbours to meet each other for the first time. We hosted these Christmas parties for the next couple of years, until our world changed with Victoria's diagnosis.

So why am I sharing about these neighbourhood Christmas parties? Not because I want to show how hospitable we were. No, rather to say that we stepped out and made ourselves vulnerable by opening up our home to people we barely knew. I remember doing the invitations and delivering them at night because I didn't want anyone to see me! We chose to sow into relationships with our neighbours, with no idea what the future held.

When Victoria was diagnosed, our neighbours were one of our key support groups. Here are some of the ways they helped us. Some offered their homes for our family and friends to stay in when they came to visit and help us out. Others came with us to Victoria's therapy appointments to look after Alexandra, who was only twelve months old at the time. Others looked after the children so Ken and I could have a night out together. A

WONDERFUL SUPPORT

few were on-call, should Victoria have a high temperature and have to go to hospital urgently. They would come and look after the other children.

A couple were on call to meet the children on the school bus, for the days the hospital appointments were delayed and we didn't make it home in time. It was such a relief to know if things were taking longer than anticipated at the hospital, or things went wrong, I could just go through a list of numbers on my phone, and keep calling people until I found someone who was able to meet the school bus. There was enough stress just trying to cope with what was happening at the hospital, without having the added stress of wondering how long the children would have to wait at the gate until we got home. What an absolute blessing these neighbours have been to us. A brilliant example of community in action.

Our experience of the church community has been the same. Our church family has been a blessing to us in many different ways. But as with our neighbours, in reflection, I can see too, how there was a season of us sowing into the church family and supporting others, followed by a season of us receiving amazing support in our time of need. And now thankfully, years later we are able to sow again into other people's lives, but now, with the benefit of our experiences, we can sow with a completely new level of compassion, love and understanding of trauma. As it says in Ecclesiastes, there is a season for everything.

VICTORIA GRACE

To everything there is a season, and a time for every matter or purpose under heaven:

A time to be born and a time to die, a time to plant and a time to pluck up what is planted,

A time to kill and a time to heal, a time to break down and a time to build up,

A time to weep and a time to laugh, a time to mourn and a time to dance,

A time to cast away stones and a time to gather stones together,

A time to embrace and a time to refrain from embracing,

A time to get and a time to lose, a time to keep and a time to cast away,

A time to rend and a time to sew, a time to keep silence and a time to speak,

A time to love and a time to hate, a time for war and a time for peace.

(Ecclesiastes 3:1-8)

WONDERFUL SUPPORT

Here is a bit more detail about the seasons of our sowing and reaping in relation to our church family. About two years before Victoria's diagnosis, a close friend's husband was diagnosed with cancer. The doctor's prognosis was not good. They had two young sons. For the eight months after his diagnosis, our family organised meal rosters, assisted with school pick-ups and drop-offs and helped out with any other practical needs. Of course we weren't the only people to come alongside this family and help, many members of our church family were helping them in many different ways. Again my reason for sharing this is not to show what we did, but rather to demonstrate the act of intentionally sowing into other people's lives in their time of need.

Who would have thought that two years later we'd have a child with cancer and be requiring a lot of practical support. Towards the end of Victoria's chemotherapy treatment, when I was literally at breaking point, our church set up a roster of people to accompany us to the hospital for her treatment appointments. It was fabulous to have the emotional support with us on those weekly visits. Church also set up a roster of people to look after our children on Saturday nights so Ken and I could get out for some much needed couple time.

In the past eighteen months, as we have entered a season of stability, we have again been able to sow into our church family, offering encouragement and support to those who find themselves in desperate family situations.

VICTORIA GRACE

This season has been a blessing for us in so many ways, especially as we can see God using all that has happened to us in the past six years, for His purposes.

I pray that as you have read these examples of community in action, you can see that community can be a wonderful thing, particularly when you are going through a crisis. But to be part of community, often you have to be vulnerable enough to make the first move to create a relationship, or even start a community. Everyone has a deep need to belong. When we are in community we can laugh together, cry together and support each other. We don't know what ups and downs our future holds, but when you are in a community it is much easier to get through each season. And of course there is the great blessing of being able to help others in their time of need.

Chapter 10

Scans and A Big Scare

EMAILS FROM 1ST OCT TO 16TH NOV 2012

EMAIL SENT ON 1ST OCTOBER 2012

This morning we waved good-bye to two very excited girls, as Charlotte and Victoria left Newcastle bound for Lake Burrendong Sport and Recreation Centre, near Wellington and Dubbo, about four hours away, on the Camp Quality Junior Camp. They each have an adult companion looking after them. They will return of Friday, no doubt full of stories and probably quite tired. Again we are so grateful for the opportunities provided for our family through this wonderful organisation.

How is Victoria going? Well, we just don't know. Her left eyelid is drooping. According to the ophthalmologist we saw last week, this could be a weak muscle problem, possibly caused by the tumour. However, there appears to be no degradation with her walking or left arm and hand use, for which we are thankful to God. So we continue to wait for the results of next week's scan.

The occupational therapist has arranged for Victoria to attend a 'school starters' class at the hospital every Monday morning of Term Four. The goal is to help her improve some of the fine motor skills required for writing, cutting etc. We are so blessed by the amazing medical support we have had and continue to receive.

It has been great to have two weeks break from the chemotherapy schedule, and try to enjoy some 'normal' family life. Although once again as the scan draws nearer, some days it is more difficult to stay positive regarding the outcome. God's word is a constant source of strength and a reminder that He is in control.

> *I will praise the LORD at all times. I will constantly speak his praises. I will boast only in the LORD; let all who are discouraged take heart. Come, let us tell of the LORD's greatness; let us exalt his name together.* (Psalm 34:1-3 NIV)

Thank you for your continued prayer and practical support.

EMAIL SENT ON 11TH OCTOBER 2012

We received the results of Victoria's MRI on Tuesday and they are very encouraging. The tumour has reduced in size since commencing the chemotherapy. We thank God for His grace and mercy.

SCANS AND A BIG SCARE

This result has given us renewed hope for complete healing for every aspect of Victoria's body, including the left eye lid drooping, and extremely limited left field vision, which both remain a mystery at this point in time.

The chemotherapy treatment will continue until July 2013, on a schedule of weekly treatments for four weeks and then two weeks off. This new schedule will start next week. The next scan will be in three months.

> *Praise be to the LORD, for he has heard my cry for mercy. The LORD is my strength and my shield; my heart trusts in him, and I am helped. My heart leaps for joy and I will give thanks to him in song.* (Psalm 28:6-7 NIV)

Words really cannot express what we are feeling after hearing this result today and our deep-felt gratitude to you all for your prayers and continuing support.

We continue to claim Victoria's namesake over her life – Victoria – conquer, victory; Grace – favour, blessing.

Victoria celebrated her fifth birthday yesterday and we look forward to her celebrating many more.

EMAIL SENT ON 2ND NOVEMBER 2012

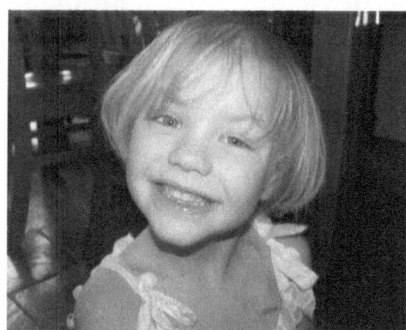

Victoria at home 24 hours after the anaphylactic reaction

To those who have been praying for us in the past 24 hours, thank you. Your covering was very much needed, as Victoria had an anaphylactic reaction, a severe immune reaction mediated by excessive histamine release, to one of the chemotherapy drugs yesterday.

Thankfully we were still in the hospital's oncology day unit just nearing the end of the day's treatment, when the reaction started. The intensive care team of about ten people were on the scene within minutes of the call being made. Needless to say it was extremely traumatic for both Victoria and me. For me, it bought back many memories of the disturbing twenty-four hours Victoria spent in the Intensive Care Unit after the brain surgery.

Victoria was kept in hospital for the night to ensure that all was indeed well. And it was. Praise be to God. Once again we are grateful for the most wonderful professional care we received at the John Hunter Hospital. This Psalm sums up the many thoughts that ran through my mind last night as we went to sleep in the hospital.

> *On my bed I remember you; I think of you through the watches of the night. Because you are my help, I sing in the shadow of your wings. My soul clings to you; your right hand upholds me.* (Psalm 63:6-8 NIV)

We are grateful too for the support team that is forming to help out with the rest of the family during such emergencies. With each experience we are discovering better strategies and reducing the level of emotional stress throughout the family, which is a priority, as I feel this journey is really only just beginning.

One of our main prayer points now is wisdom for the doctors regarding Victoria's treatment. Some adjustment to the current treatment will be necessary and thankfully there are some options. Please pray that they decide on the best treatment.

Thank you again for your prayers and continued support.

EMAIL SENT ON 9TH NOVEMBER 2012

Life continues to be a rollercoaster of emotions; this week thankfully, mostly joy.

Wednesday morning was Victoria's kindergarten

orientation, the first year of formal schooling. I was a little bit nervous about who her teacher would be, as Victoria will face some challenges physically and miss at least one day of school each week for treatment. Clearly I should have been trusting God a bit more on this, because when we arrived at school and as I looked in the window of the kindergarten room I saw two of the most beautiful teachers, both of whom we already have great relationships with. The tears started to flow and they didn't stop until half way through the morning. I felt so loved by God, and so reassured of His love and provision for Victoria. Victoria herself had no tears, and absolutely loved the morning and is so keen to start kindergarten.

Thank you for your prayers regarding Victoria's change in treatment. Victoria's oncologist has decided to put her on a different chemotherapy drug, to avoid last week's reaction happening again. So we are on weekly visits with no breaks for the next 6 weeks. The next scan is scheduled for 29th January, the day before she starts kindergarten.

God has taught me many things on this journey so far, including greater compassion for those who have on-going illnesses, either physically or mentally. However one of the biggest lessons has been learning how to live with the fact that we do not know what is going to confront us from day to day. My profession prior to having children involved project planning and risk management to the nth degree at both St George Bank and Westpac's head offices in Sydney. So I find it rather ironic that I am in the

SCANS AND A BIG SCARE

situation now where any day can be turned completely upside down and requires minute by minute trusting and calling on God for wisdom and peace. Clearly all the skills I learnt in the corporate sphere were for a far greater purpose than helping improve their efficiency.

Thank you again for your continuing prayer and support.

> *God remembered us when we were down, His love never quits. Rescued us from the trampling boot, His love never quits. Takes care of everyone in time of need, His love never quits. Thank God, who did it all! His love never quits.* (Psalm 136:23-26 The Message)

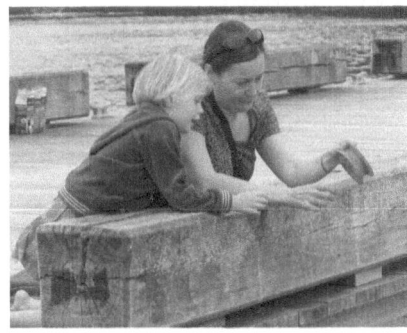

Keeping life as normal as possible, fishing with a faithful friend who has been alongside us on this journey from the beginning

EMAIL SENT ON 16 NOVEMBER 2012

This is just a quick update to let you know that Victoria was unable to have chemotherapy, vinblastine, yesterday because her neutrophil count was too low, meaning her immunity is currently very low. Her doctor is considering reducing the dose next week. Within herself, Victoria is well, just a bit more tired than normal.

We would appreciate specific prayer for her well-being at this time of vulnerability. Thank you.

Scripture for the day:

> *For everything that was written in the past was written to teach us, so that through the endurance taught in the Scriptures and the encouragement they provide we might have hope.* (Romans 15:4 NIV)

What more is there to say other than Amen!

REFLECTION – PLAN B PREPARING FOR THE CRISIS

When Victoria had an anaphylactic reaction to one of the chemotherapy drugs, resulting in an unplanned stay in hospital, my priority after Victoria's well-being, was the happenings at home. It was one of those days when I went through the list of neighbours on my phone until I could find someone who could meet the children at the bus stop and look after them until Ken returned from work. A phone call to school was required to let the children know of the change of plan, and try as best as possible to not cause panic in them regarding their sister's health. Basically it was, put Plan B into action.

> *Plan B, the contingency plan, consisted of four parts: communications; hospital admission; home arrangements and homecoming. We also had to use Plan B when Victoria became febrile, with a temperature higher than 38 degrees Celsius, at home and so was required to go to hospital asap. Appendix E has a master list of all the lists that make up Plan B.*

PLAN B

Communications

There were five groups of people that I had to communicate with at this time, our prayer warriors, our children, the school teachers, our home helpers and our hospital helpers.

Activating the prayer chain was one of the first things I did when things started to go awry during a hospital visit. I believe strongly in the power of prayer. I had a group our prayer warrior's contact numbers set up in my phone. Throughout the crisis, I always tried to keep them updated, and always let them know when our prayers had been answered. In our journey there have been many testimonies of God's faithfulness, and I believe this encourages others to call on His name in their time of tribulation.

> *Confess your trespasses to one another, and pray for one another, that you may be healed. The effective, fervent prayer of a righteous man avails much.* (James 5:16 NKJV)

Reminding our other children about the contingency plan was a key component to reducing the anxiety levels at home in the times of an unplanned hospital admission. On chemotherapy treatment days, before Marshall and Charlotte got on the school bus I would remind them that

SCANS AND A BIG SCARE

Victoria was having treatment today and that all going well, we would be home from the hospital before they got home from school. But if there was a delay, I would contact the school and give them a message regarding the change of plans.

Communication with the school teachers was also an important part of the plan. If Victoria was in hospital, no matter what plans I put in place for home, it would always be different without mummy being there. Sometimes, stress caused by this change manifested in the children's behaviour at school. So I always tried to keep the teachers informed so that they had a bit of background on what was happening at home.

Thankfully, as I mentioned in a previous chapter, we had a huge practical support group. Many of our neighbours had graciously agreed to be part of the on-call list to help out with the other children, should we be delayed at hospital or have an unplanned admission. All of their contact numbers were in my phone, ready should I need to call them. I also had a laminated sheet with their numbers on it, just in-case my phone ran out of battery. I quickly learnt to put my phone charger in my hospital emergency bag.

As the months of chemotherapy treatment went by, I realised we needed to make provision for our emotional well-being during these hospital stays. Normally by the second day Victoria was feeling a lot better, and was keen to go home. However, Victoria was required to stay for three days, until it was confirmed that there was nothing growing on the blood cultures that were taken when she was admitted to hospital. So we put together a list of people we could ask to visit us in hospital. Some of these people would sit with Victoria so I could have a break from the hospital room. Others on the list were school friends of Victoria's who would come, sit on the bed with Victoria and play for about half an hour. It is very confronting going into a children's cancer ward, not an easy thing to do. We are very grateful for those people who did come to visit us. Their visits meant so much to us and definitely helped to break up the monotony of the day.

Unplanned Hospital Admission

Plan B included making sure that every time Victoria and I went to hospital, we were practically prepared for an unplanned hospital admission. The pre-packed Hospital overnight bags were the key part of our preparation. As unplanned admissions, particularly those associated with high temperatures, usually required at least a three day stay in hospital, we needed to pack sufficient clothes, activities and also business papers. We are grateful that hospitals in Australia provide sheets, blankets and food, unlike some other countries in the world.

> *Appendix F contains the Emergency Hospital Bag Contents Checklist. A list of the items I had in pre-packed bags for Victoria and myself in case of an emergency visit to hospital.*

Home arrangements

My goal was that Marshall, Charlotte and Alexandra would be minimally impacted by these unplanned hospital admissions. Not an easy goal to achieve, but I did my best with the help of Ken and our fantastic support team. At the time when Victoria was having chemotherapy, the children were still very young, Marshall eight, Charlotte, six and Alexandra two years old. Each child had their own fears and anxieties about their sister's health and the absence of their mum.

There were a few things I put in place to help keep things running as smoothly as possible at home.

1. **A list of sleepover options for each child.** Having one less child at home definitely made it easier for the home support person, or for Ken.

2. **Documented home routines for the morning; afternoon and evening.** These routines helped to

give the children some sense of control.

3. **Instructions for how to use the home equipment.** For example the washing machine, dishwasher and television. I'd created these checklists when Victoria was born, as my beautiful mother would come over from New Zealand and help out with Marshall and Charlotte while I tended to baby Victoria, and then two years later, to baby Alexandra.

4. **The login details online school canteen orders.** So I could order Marshall and Charlotte's lunches online, while in hospital with Victoria. Getting a lunch order from the canteen was a big treat for them, as normally they only had one lunch order a term, and a bonus one on their birthday.

5. **Registered for After School Care.** As a back-up to the contingency plan, we also had Marshall and Charlotte on the casual list for After School Care, in the event that none of our support team were available to help out after school.

Home coming

As you have probably gathered from reading through this summary of Plan B these unplanned hospital admissions are extremely disruptive, distressing and completely emotionally exhausting for each family member. So I felt it was a good idea to carefully plan the home-coming from these admissions and to celebrate that we were all home together as a family again.

> Appendix G contains the Homecoming Checklist. A list of the tasks to be done when preparing to leave the hospital and the phone calls to make on the way home in the car. It also includes activities to be done when we arrived at home to ensure everything was prepared for the next emergency hospital visit.

One of the key things about the home coming was the adjustment for Victoria and me coming back into the family environment. Our drive home from hospital always included a chat about Victoria having mummy to herself for three days, and how when we get home, mummy will need to devote some time to Marshall, Charlotte, Alexandra, and of course daddy.

Another important part of the home coming was the celebratory dinner, as you will read about in some of my emails. The dinner was normally a take away pizza courtesy of my mum and dad, as the last thing I wanted to do was cook a dinner. But more important than the food, was the conversation that was to take place, the acknowledgement that it had been a difficult few days but by the grace of God we got through, and we had many things to be thankful for. We said a prayer of thanks to our faithful God and then took turns of saying thank you to another family member, citing an example of the help they had given us.

> *It is a good thing to give thanks to the LORD, and to sing praises to Your name, O most High; to declare Your lovingkindness in the morning, and your faithfulness every night.* (Psalm 92:1-2 NKJV)

Chapter 11

The Silly Season

EMAILS FROM 26TH NOV TO 28TH DEC 2012

EMAIL SENT ON 26 NOVEMBER 2012

As Christmas approaches and I think about this past year, there is only one word that comes to mind, grace.

I cannot begin to describe the grace that God has shown us all this year. This scripture resonates within my heart,

> "But he said to me, "My grace is sufficient for you, for my power is made perfect in weakness." Therefore I will boast all the more gladly about my weaknesses, so that Christ's power may rest on me."
> (2 Corinthians 12:9-10 NIV)

Victoria continues to live her life to the full. She was able to have chemotherapy last week as her neutrophil count had improved.

It appears as though Victoria has almost no left field vision as a result of the brain surgery. So we met with Vision

Australia last week to learn about training strategies and safety in relation to this loss. Previously we had thought that if she bumped into something it was due to unsteadiness on her feet due to the left side weakness, however now we know she just couldn't see it. So if you are ever walking with her, please walk on her left. If you feel led to pray for a miracle with her eyesight, please do.

We have had a weekend filled with the blessing of God, through the generosity of two amazing organisations.

On Saturday we participated in an event organised by the Starlight Children's Foundation. We caught the Starlight Express, a decorated XPT train, from Sydney central station to Thirlmere, a one and half hour journey. The train was filled with Starlight Children's Foundation staff, volunteers and Countrylink volunteers. Even the train driver had volunteered his time. They all made the journey lots of fun, with morning tea, balloon animals, colouring competitions and chats with the Captain Starlight's who normally work at the Children's hospitals. When we arrived at the TrainWorks Park at Thirlmere, we were greeted by another dedicated lot of volunteers who provided masses of entertainment, including face painting, which Alexandra loved, and lunch. We all had a wonderful time, Ken was especially pleased as he got to see the train round house in action with a steam train. We returned to Central by the XPT, half of the travellers asleep with exhaustion, the other half on a sugar rush after the "treats" eaten throughout the day.

It was an excellent family day, giving us all an opportunity to "get away" from all the challenges for a day, and just have fun.

On Sunday we were treated to another wonderful afternoon at the Camp Quality Christmas party at the Leisure Centre at Raymond Terrace. Once again we were able to relax and just enjoy some time out. It is also good, well, in some ways, to be with other families who have or are going through similar experiences to us. Victoria had fun in the pool with a little girl the same age as her, who is often sitting in the chair next to her on Thursdays having chemotherapy. It was wonderful to see them both laughing and running around in the pool together, knowing they shared a common bond that is rather uncommon.

Thank you again for your wonderful prayers and support. I hope you don't mind that I have shared about our experiences this weekend, it is just that I am still constantly amazed by the love shown to our family in so many different ways, including these great organisations, their volunteers and financial supporters.

EMAIL SENT ON 29TH NOVEMBER 2012

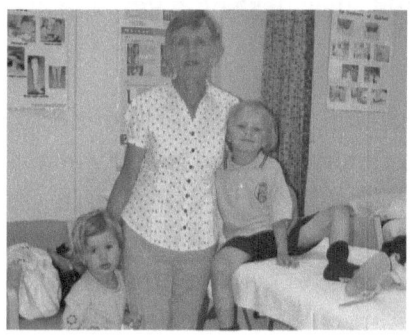

Alexandra, Granny Bett and Victoria in the Physiotherapy Department at John Hunter Children's Hospital

Just a quick update today. Thanks for your continuing prayers, Victoria was well enough to have chemotherapy today.

We have had my wonderful mother, visiting from NZ, here for the last 2 weeks, helping out with absolutely everything! One of the best things about this visit, is that we are not currently in 'crisis' mode, so we have had quite a few times when we can just sit and chat, something that hasn't happened for 2 years. Of course there have been a couple of hospital visits, including the one in the photos, where Victoria is having a mould made for a new splint. Victoria has requested that this splint is purple with butterflies on it, so we will see what turns up in a couple of weeks.

One specific prayer point is that the side-effects of the chemotherapy that Victoria is currently having are kept to a minimum.

Thank you again for your prayers and support.

> *The LORD gives strength to his people;*
> *the LORD blesses his people with peace.*
> (Psalm 29:11 NIV)

EMAIL SENT ON 2ND DECEMBER 2012

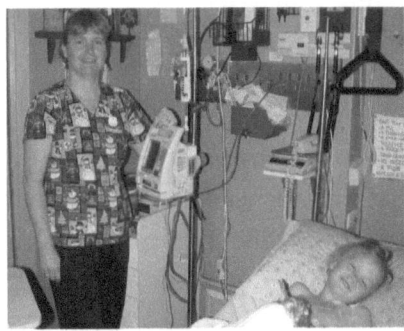

Nurse and Victoria at John Hunter Children's Hospital, J1 ward

As some of you already know, Victoria was admitted to hospital yesterday with a high temperature. After prayer and antibiotics she is looking a lot brighter today. She will remain in hospital until at least tomorrow.

It is all rather festive in ward J1, with the nursing staff wearing special Christmas shirts, and the corridors are decorated with tinsel and lights. Marshall helped to put the fairy lights around the door of Victoria's room.

Many, many thanks to everyone who has helped to make this hospital visit so easy. Now even these emergency hospital visits are becoming normal to our family. How bizarre life is.

> *Oh, give thanks to the LORD, for He is good! For His mercy endures forever.*
> (1 Chronicles 16:34 NKJV)

Thank you again for your continuing prayer and practical support. Both are absolutely vital to us.

EMAIL SENT ON 3RD DECEMBER 2012

Victoria was given the all clear to come home this morning, praise God. Yesterday Victoria was well enough to have a couple of friends from Prep visit her in hospital, which provided short spurts of much needed entertainment. It is great to see that God has blessed her by surrounding her with compassionate and caring friends at such a young age.

Thanks again for all your prayers and support.

EMAIL SENT ON 9TH DECEMBER 2012

Victoria was well enough to have chemo last Thursday, and with the help of a wonderful friend who came to sit with Victoria at the hospital, I was able to attend an award presentation for Charlotte at school. It meant the world to Charlotte to see both her mum and dad at the presentation supporting her.

THE SILLY SEASON

On Friday Victoria was suffering from bad headaches and her eyes were very sensitive to light, we couldn't have the light on in the room, so off to the John Hunter Hospital we went late Friday night. Victoria was given some pain relief which fixed the headaches and some Phenergan to help the eyes, assuming it was an allergic reaction to something. By Sunday morning she was well enough to leave the hospital, and had a stop off in the Santa seat as we left the J1 ward. Ken did a great job looking after Marshall, Charlotte and Alexandra, with the help of some more wonderful friends, help for which we are very grateful.

While in hospital I had plenty of time to think about the impact of these hospital visits on our family, and think about ways to reduce the time it takes us to return to 'normal' when Victoria returns home. One idea I came up with initiated by something I read in an excellent book called, Growing Great Girls [19], was to have a special dinner, involving take-away pizza, to celebrate the homecoming and a 'round the dinner table' discussion where each family member thanks another family member for a specific thing they have done to help make the time away from each other easier. And so that is exactly what we did tonight, and it was a great success.

After some more reflection I have realised that it is currently taking about sixty people providing varying practical and emotional support to keep our family afloat, and that does not include all the faithful people praying for us, nor all the amazing medical staff. This provision from God is astonishing.

It is so true,

> The LORD will guide you always; he will satisfy your needs in a sun-scorched land and will strengthen your frame. You will be like a well-watered garden, like a spring whose waters never fail. (Isaiah 58:11 NIV)

Thank you again for your continued support, please be encouraged. We are tired, but we know God is in the midst.

EMAIL SENT ON 15TH DECEMBER 2012

I am glad to report that we are at home today, no additional hospital visits this weekend, Hallelujah! And no side effects to be seen this week. Another Hallelujah. Thanks to everyone who has been storming heaven on our behalf.

This week has been filled with blessings for Victoria and our family, including a very festive day at the John Hunter Hospital on Thursday, with visits by the Hunter Valley Zoo, some of the Newcastle Jets soccer team, Captain Starlight, Santa and Mrs Clause. We then arrived home to a beautiful hamper, generously given to us by a friend's church. Tuesday night we were given a tour of Newcastle in a stretch hummer, courtesy of Camp Quality.

THE SILLY SEASON

Victoria received her new splint on Monday, purple with butterflies, just as she had ordered. The physio has advised that her calf and hamstring muscles are tightening, so we now have a regime of leg stretches to do each day. This will be reviewed in mid-January.

Of course Wednesday was Victoria's last day at Prep, another milestone in her life. We are grateful to God that she has probably only missed four days of Prep because of ill health since starting chemo and pray that this good health will continue in 2013 and beyond.

This is the scripture I have written on my kitchen whiteboard this morning:

> *Shouts of joy and victory resound in the tents of the righteous: The LORD's right hand has done mighty things!* (Psalm 118:15 NIV)

Amen!

Thank you again for your continued prayer and support. We pray you are enjoying the festive season.

EMAIL SENT ON 20TH DECEMBER 2012

Victoria was unable to have chemotherapy today as her neutrophil count was too low. The next chemotherapy treatment is scheduled for Thursday 27th December.

Can you please pray that:

- ♥ The neutrophils grow quickly so her immune system can be restored

- ♥ Victoria will not have to be in hospital on Christmas Day

Charlotte accompanied us to the hospital today and was a wonderful help, reading stories to Victoria and helping her with various craft activities. One of the beautiful nurses in the day unit took extra time to explain each step in the process to Charlotte, including showing us the automatic shoot that takes the blood samples to the pathology department. It was good to be able to take some of the 'mystery' out of the hospital 'goings-on' for Charlotte.

Thanks again for your prayers and support.

EMAIL SENT ON 25TH DECEMBER 2012

Thank you for your prayers, praise God we are all at home for Christmas. We have all had a lovely morning with Ken's parents, sister and niece.

One of the biggest blessings of 2012 is that every member of our family has finished the year in a much better state emotionally than when the year started. Thank you to everyone who has contributed this year to our emotional well-being, whether it has been via an encouraging email, a chat at the front gate, school or church, a gift, practical help of some sort, prayer, a hug, a smile or a wave. We praise God that you are all in our lives.

> *Then that person can pray to God and find favour with him, they will see God's face and shout for joy; he will restore them to full well-being.* (Job 33:26 NIV)

Merry Christmas to you and your family

PS: Ken's aunt has faithfully made us a chocolate cake every month this year, and we used the December cake as a birthday cake for Jesus.

EMAIL SENT ON 28TH DECEMBER 2012

Victoria's neutrophils were up to 0.7 yesterday so she was able to have chemotherapy, the cut-off is 0.5. Charlotte accompanied us again to the hospital and was a great help, feeling quite at home, talking with the doctors and nurses.

Victoria is good today, not too tired and very pleased with herself in that every day this week she has swum in the pool without her bubble on. The headaches that were so prevalent a few weeks ago have gone.

I met with the Ronald McDonald Learning Program liaison person yesterday, at the hospital. Her role is to help to ensure that Victoria doesn't fall behind with her schooling due to the days off school for treatment and illness. She will liaise with us and the school until Victoria finishes Year Twelve. The initial help, funded by the Ronald McDonald House Charities, will be a tutor for one hour a week for forty weeks. Once again I was overwhelmed with this level of support provided at no cost to us.

Thanks again for your prayers and I pray you are all enjoying a post-Christmas rest.

> *But let all who take refuge in you be glad; let them ever sing for joy. Spread your protection over them, that those who love your name may rejoice in you. For surely, O LORD, you bless the righteous; you surround them with your favour as with a shield.*
> (Psalm 5:11-12 NIV)

THE SILLY SEASON

REFLECTION – MOTHERS

Mothers. Precious mothers. Where to start? I asked the Holy Spirit and thankfully He showed me exactly how to start this reflection, with a beautiful poem by Helen Steiner Rice [20]

A MOTHER'S LOVE

A Mother's love is something that no one can explain,
It is made of deep devotion and of sacrifice and pain,
It is endless and unselfish and enduring come what may
For nothing can destroy it or take that love away ...
It is patient and forgiving when all others are forsaking,
And it never fails or falters even though the heart is breaking ...
It believes beyond believing when the world around condemns

And it glows with all the beauty of the rarest, brightest gems ...
It is far beyond defining, it defies all explanation,
And it still remains a secret like the mysteries of creation ...

VICTORIA GRACE

> *A many splendored miracle man cannot understand*
> *And another wondrous evidence of God's tender guiding hand.*

This poem describes perfectly the love my mother has given me, especially lines like

> *It is endless and unselfish and enduring come what may...*

> *And it never fails or falters even though the heart is breaking*

A friend visiting from interstate at the same time my mother was staying with us said something like this of my mother,

'Wendy, your mum is amazing. You can see it isn't easy for her to be here with all the pain and suffering Victoria is going through, but she has a determination about her, that even though it isn't easy for her, she is going to be here no matter what.'

That was a very accurate observation. It can't be easy to see your daughter's family in crisis mode with your granddaughter seriously ill. But my mother was determined to do whatever she could do to help. The Redkite organisation acknowledges the impact a grandchild's cancer diagnosis has on the grandparents.

THE SILLY SEASON

When a child suffers from cancer, their whole family is affected. Studies show that grandparents often carry an emotional burden which is two-fold: for their children and their grandchildren... From the devastating moment of diagnosis, grandparents often play a significant caring and practical support role in their families. [21]

Redkite provides a telesupport group for grandparents living in Australia. Ken's parents have participated in one of these groups.

I think about my mum and how it must have been for her when I phoned that night just after 2am New Zealand time, and told her what the neurologist had just told me. My mum knew I had taken Victoria to the hospital, but like Ken and me, she had no idea that this diagnosis was likely. I can't imagine how it was for her, hearing that news from me. She showed me so much love and grace when I didn't even ask if she could come and help. I just said, 'Mum, I need you.' And she literally caught the first flight out of Auckland to Sydney and then made the two and half hour trip up to Newcastle.

My first phone call that night of course had been to Ken, who was in Melbourne on a business trip. I had asked the neurologist to speak with him, as I just couldn't tell him. I knew that I didn't have the emotional strength to cope with his reaction to the news. Thankfully, the neurologist did a brilliant job talking with him. As soon as the call with Ken was finished, I phoned my mum. I know that Ken then phoned his mum too, and was talking to her for a significant part of the night. Praise God for mums who make themselves available to their children.

Over these three years my Mum has often visited us, providing practical and emotional support. Initially her visits were around scan times, and then for various periods during Victoria's chemotherapy treatment.

This journey has been uncharted waters for us all. Our lives had been touched by cancer before with extended family and friends, but not directly with a child. As we bumbled our way through each day, learning how to love and care for each other in this new constantly changing environment, there was plenty of scope for a complete breakdown of our relationship. There have been moments of exhaustion, leading to misunderstandings and tears. But they have always been resolved, if not straight away, normally after a good night's sleep for all concerned. Praise God for His wisdom in creating day and night, and His promise that His mercies are new every morning.

> *The steadfast love of the Lord never ceases; his mercies never come to an end; they are new every morning; great is your faithfulness.* (Lamentations 3:22-23 ESV)

I am so grateful for the way my mother has loved me, with an encouraging love that affirms me in the difficult moments, and a practical love that always looks for ways to help. She has taught me, more through actions than words, how to be a generous mum, a mum who doesn't give up and that hangs in there with her children, no matter how tough it gets. Those life lessons have given me the foundations to be the mother I have needed to be to our children as we continue on through these uncharted waters.

Ken's mother has been a wonderful support to him too. Always being a listening ear as he tried to make sense of what is happening with his daughter. She has also been a great practical support to me, especially in the first six months of Victoria's chemotherapy treatment. Living only forty-five minutes away from us, Ken's mum and dad came to our home each week to look after Alexandra while I took Victoria to the hospital for treatment. Not only did Ken's mum look after Alexandra, but she cleaned our home. It was a huge blessing for me to know that Alexandra was being well cared for and that our home was a cleaner environment, reducing the risk of infection for Victoria.

I am blessed to have a mother and a mother-in-law who value family so highly, and have been great role models for their children. We are blessed that they have been fit, well and available to help us in our time of great need. I realise this is not always the case for other families, so have tried to not take their help for granted.

VICTORIA GRACE

Under the guidance of the Holy Spirit, I am finishing this reflection with another of Helen Steiner Rice's poems.

A MOTHER'S DAY PRAYER [22]

"Our Father in Heaven whose love is divine,
Thanks for the love of a Mother like mine –
And in Thy great mercy look down from above
And grant this dear Mother the gift of Your love –
And all through the year, whatever betide her,
Assure her each day that You are beside her –
And, Father in Heaven, show me the way
To lighten her tasks and brighten her day,
And bless her dear heart with the insight to see
That her love means more than the world to me."

Chapter 12

New Year and a Blog

EMAILS FROM 6TH JAN TO 24TH JAN 2013

EMAIL SENT ON 6TH JANUARY 2013

Wow, we have made it to 2013. Happy New Year!

For us the start of a new year has more significance than ever before. We praise God that He has given us the strength and grace to travel another twelve months on this road. And thank Him with the expectation that in 2013 He will do the same.

Victoria is doing very well. She is now on a schedule of three weeks on Thursday treatments and one week off. Last Thursday was an off week and it was wonderful to spend the day at home as a family.

Tomorrow we are off for a week's holiday at Harry's House at Stockton. Harry's House is a retreat for families with children living with cancer, or for families grieving the loss of a child to cancer within the past two years. The retreat has been established by an amazing family, David

& Samantha Meyn of East Maitland. Their son, Harry at the age of six, was diagnosed with a brain tumour and sadly passed away seven months after diagnosis.

The establishment and availability of this retreat is a huge blessing to us, as we really can't be further than 1 hours' drive from the hospital. Also Victoria is scheduled for chemotherapy treatment this week, so we will need to make the trip to the John Hunter Hospital on Thursday. We are looking forward to days at the beach in the sand and surf.

I have a few prayer points for anyone who feels led to pray for us:

- That Victoria will be able to complete the next three weeks of treatment without any issues, which will mean she can attend the first three days of kindergarten without any interruptions

- That God's peace will reign over us as we come to the two year milestone from Victoria's initial diagnosis, and that there will be time for any grief to surface and be processed well. By 'grief' I mean the loss of expectations as to how our family would be and what we would be doing now. Of course we are so very grateful to God and the grace and favour He has given us during the past two years, however that does not negate the fact that two years ago we certainly did not expect to be in the midst of these circumstances.

- ♥ That God's peace will reign over us as Victoria's next scan approaches on January 29th, with the hope that the vinblastine is doing the same or better job than the previous chemotherapy.

> *The LORD is my strength and my shield; my heart trusts in him and I am helped. My heart leaps for joy and I will give him thanks in song.* (Psalm 28:7 NIV)

Thank you again for your continued prayer and support.

EMAIL SENT ON 11TH JANUARY 2013

We have had four great days at Harry's House so far. It is a beautiful house, an absolute retreat. I cried for about an hour when we arrived here, overwhelmed by the generosity and thoughtfulness of everyone who has contributed to this house. Meanwhile the children ran from room to room checking out all the appointments and reporting back that every bedroom had a TV and DVD player - what a treat.

It has been so good to get away and have a break from 'normal' life. Although it is clear that this retreat has been built with a specific group of people in mind. In one of the kitchen cupboards are the stunning purple plastic gloves, vomit bags and lots of medicine measuring cups and syringes.

VICTORIA GRACE

Yesterday we went on a family outing to the John Hunter Hospital for Victoria's chemotherapy. The adventure started with all the children watching Victoria's port being accessed, and then watching the containers of blood go up the shoot to the pathology department.

While waiting for the blood test results, we went to see the physiotherapist. Victoria's splint has been hurting in a couple of places so she has not been wearing it for the past week. Not having the splint on makes a huge difference to both Victoria's gait and confidence.

The physio advised that the problem is with the tightening of Victoria's leg muscles, most likely due to less activity, as she has been more resting due to tiredness, and the chemotherapy. So the physio made a boot for each leg for Victoria to wear at night time to give both legs a good stretch.

Victoria thought she would like different coloured boots for each leg.

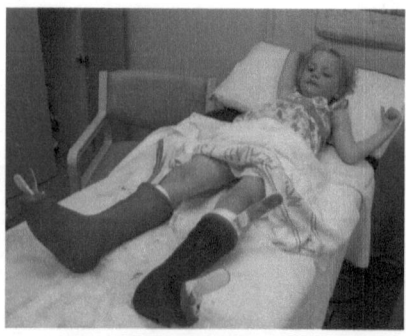

Victoria getting night splints made in the Physiotherapy Department at John Hunter Hospital

However, we only took the left boot home with us, as the right one didn't quite have the correct stretch position. Next week we will visit the physio again and try the splint on, to see if Victoria's foot and leg are better positioned in it. Possibly the physio will have another attempt at making a night boot for the right leg.

After the night boots were made, we went back to the Day Unit. Victoria's blood test results were good. She was able to have the chemotherapy.

After the treatment we visited the fairy garden and the Starlight Express Room. The girls had a fun time making lots of crafts with Captain Starlight and the volunteers. Captain Starlight gave them each a woollen doll that had been made by some local high school students. Marshall had fun playing with all the electronic gadgets.

All in all it was a very successful hospital visit, with every family member getting more appreciation of what Victoria goes through each week, and the challenges she faces.

A specific prayer point this week is that Victoria's leg muscles will stretch as required with the use of the night boots and the daily stretching regime.

Here is an encouraging scripture I read this week.

> *God can do anything, you know - far more than you could ever imagine or guess or*

request in your wildest dreams! He does it not by pushing us around but by working within us, his Spirit deeply and gently within us. (Ephesians 3:20a The Message)

Thank you again for your prayers and continued support as we continue to trust God with Victoria.

EMAIL SENT ON 17TH JANUARY 2013

When Victoria was initially in hospital two years ago, and I was sending out my first Victoria Update email, one of the nurses said to me, 'Some of the mums do blogs to keep people updated.'

I politely replied, 'Oh really', thinking to myself that Victoria will be out of here soon and that will be the end of it.

Well it seems that this has not been the case, probably an understatement. So guess what, I have created a blog as a way of communicating what is happening with Victoria. The blog is at victoriagraceconqueror.blogspot.com.au

I hope you enjoy reading through the blog, and are encouraged by the testimony of our Lord's faithfulness, as we ourselves are so encouraged each day.

Thank you again for your prayers and support.

BLOG POST ON 17TH JANUARY 2013

Victoria was able to have chemotherapy today, despite her neutrophils being a bit low. Charlotte came up to the hospital and was an awesome support.

The girls did some craft and played with their Barbie dolls during the treatment. At this point in time Victoria is on track to have treatment next week and then will have an off week, the first week of school. This will be such a blessing. She is so excited about school.

We also had another visit to the physio. The review showed that the night boot had stretched Victoria's muscles sufficiently that she can now wear her AFO again. Another Praise God! Thank you to everyone who was praying for this specific healing.

The physio made another night boot for the right leg, to help those muscles stretch out too.

PRAYER POINTS

- ♥ The chemotherapy will continue to shrink the tumour

- ♥ Victoria will be well enough to attend the first three days of kindergarten

- ♥ The night boots will continue to stretch her muscles sufficiently

We are feeling confident about the next scan on 29th January, trusting that God has it all under control.

> *Ah, Sovereign LORD, you have made the heavens and the earth by your great power and outstretched arm. Nothing is too hard for you. (Jeremiah 32:17 NIV)*

We thank God that as we approach the two year anniversary since Victoria's diagnosis, she is well and enjoying every aspect of her life. She even graduated to the next swimming class this week. Victoria Grace, you truly are a conqueror in God's strength.

Thank you again for your continuing prayers and support.

BLOG POST ON 24TH JANUARY 2013

We thank God that Victoria was able to have chemo yesterday so she can now attend the first three days of school next week.

During an appointment with the OT this week, Victoria did another school readiness assessment. The assessment showed improvement in her motor-planning regarding writing, pencil grip and paper cutting, which is all very positive. She also provided some helpful hints for Victoria in the class room. One hint was to put stickers in the left hand margin of the page to help Victoria find the left hand side of the page due to the field vision loss. Without the stickers, Victoria starts to write about half way across the left page.

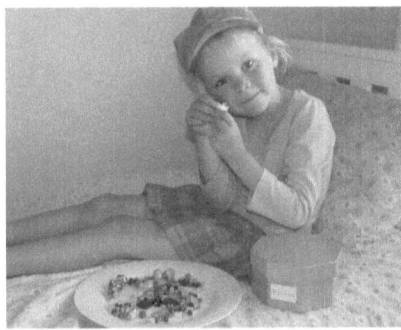

Victoria at home with her bravery beads

At the end of each hospital visit, the nurses give Victoria, and siblings if they are there, bravery beads for various events that have taken place. For example: Green beads for clinic visits; Purple beads for Chemotherapy treatment; Stars for port accessing; and WOW beads for being fantastic. These beads provide encouragement to the children and acknowledge what they have done on each hospital visit. Currently the bravery beads are safely stored in some beautiful boxes given to us by one of the very thoughtful school teachers. They take pride of place in the kitchen. Some of the mums have embroidered them on to calico teddy bears or quilts. We are not sure what we will do with ours at this stage.

Charlotte once again accompanied us to the hospital and was wonderful support. I decided to reward her diligence and thoughtfulness towards her sister by letting her buy a piece of clothing. Charlotte has been an absolute blessing to Victoria on these hospital visits, keeping her entertained and showing compassion when the various procedures are being done. I believe the experiences of these hospital visits and the understanding she has gained, will help her to cope with the challenges that lie ahead this year.

During the past couple of weeks Victoria has started to ask questions. Why am I the only one in our family who has a port? Why am I the only one who has to do chemotherapy? Why am I the only one who has to wear a splint?

My response was, 'I don't know why you are the only one in our family who has to go through these things. But God has given you all you need to deal with this. He knows you can cope with it.'

I then went on to explain to Victoria that I send emails to people asking them to pray for her. She was very pleased about that. We then sat down and together looked through a book I have created for her with all the photos that I have attached to the emails, and printed out comments and scriptures that people have emailed or texted in relation to her courage and bravery. The purpose of this was to remind Victoria of all the things she has already overcome, and of all the people who are praying for her, and of the immense love of her Heavenly Father.

I thank God for the wisdom and foresight God gave me

in putting this book together late last year, knowing that the extra encouragement was going to be needed as Victoria's world view widens.

I believe that this scripture is going to be a key one for Victoria in the coming months and years.

> *No test or temptation that comes your way is beyond the course of what others have had to face. All you need to remember is that God will never let you down, he'll never let you be pushed past your limit, he'll always be there to help you through it.*
> (1 Corinthians 10:13 The Message)

Thank you for your continuing prayers and support, particularly as Victoria has the MRI next week and we receive the results on Wednesday 6th February. We continue to thank God for all He has done, all He is doing, and all He is going to do.

VICTORIA GRACE

REFLECTION – WRITING AS THERAPY

From the beginning of this journey, my writing has played a central role. At first I was hurriedly writing in notebooks as doctors spoke to us about what was happening with Victoria. I wanted to make sure I recorded every word they said, so we could review it later and prepare questions for our next meeting. I am so grateful for those notebooks, as they have been an invaluable record and enabled me to write about those first couple of weeks in such great detail.

About ten days after Victoria's diagnosis, as the initial crisis subsided, I began writing emails from hospital to family and friends. I sent news of Victoria's health and specific prayer requests, once, sometimes twice a day. This method of communication helped to dramatically reduce the number of phone calls we received. While I appreciate that people were concerned and wanted to know how we were going, for me constantly repeating the updates became very emotionally draining. The single email communication also gave me more time to process what was happening, and focus on helping Victoria feel safe.

Emailing an update to family and friends also meant that when I saw them or talked to them, we could chat about the more normal aspects of life. I could hear more about what was going on in their lives. This outward focus helped me to keep in touch with others, rather than getting consumed with our family's circumstances.

NEW YEAR AND A BLOG

I didn't want to be talking about our situation, especially the negative aspects, in front of our children, particularly Victoria. Our children knew what was going on, but I felt they didn't need to be constantly reminded of their sister's illness and the impact it was having on all of us.

During those initial weeks in hospital, a nurse told me that parents often write a blog aimed at updating family and friends on the child's well-being. At the time, I dismissed the idea, as I thought our experience with cancer would be over in a few months. How wrong I was.

In late 2012, when Victoria was having chemotherapy, I began to think about blogging and its benefits, in keeping family and friends updated. It would provide a single place where people could follow our story, rather than flicking back through emails, if they wanted to know the history of our journey. The blog would also enable me to publish more photos without consuming people's download quotas. And as we all know, a picture tells a thousand words.

The Christmas holidays in 2012 seemed like the perfect time to set up the blog. A few weeks free of school and work commitments meant I had plenty of time to build it.

Blogging was not new to me. In 2010 I had started a blog about our family sailing experiences, Cruising Family Robinson. We were planning to sail from Lake Macquarie, NSW to the Whitsundays, QLD, in mid-2011. The blog was to be a record of our preparation, as well as our voyage. However, one day when we were doing some coastal sailing, a shakedown (practice) cruise, things went a little awry, requiring us to get the assistance of Marine Rescue. We took this as a sign that God didn't want us to undertake the voyage at this time. Our decision was confirmed a few months later when Victoria was diagnosed.

However, even though the voyage was off, I had gained some experience and confidence with blogging, another example of how God prepares us for the future without our realising it. So with that blogging experience, I went about setting up the Victoria Grace Conqueror blog. I didn't need a complicated high powered blogging system. I only needed a vehicle that would help me to get my story out there. The free service, Blogger, suited my needs perfectly.

Writing the blog gave me a way of communicating additional information other than the state of Victoria's health and our prayer requests. One of my goals with the blog was to give people a fuller picture of what it is like to be a family living with a child with cancer. For example it allowed me to include a page of information about the charities that supported families like ours.

Having a child who is seriously ill, especially in a large family, means we needed a lot of help to 'keep all the balls in the air.' Sometimes I was tired of having to continually ask people for help. Two and a half years is a long time to be very dependent on other people for your family's well-being. I found that blogging about some of the daily struggles and being honest about how I was coping, gave me a way of indirectly asking for help. Often, after writing about a difficult week, I would get texts or emails from family and friends, either encouraging me or offering to help in some practical way. For example, doing my shopping, hanging out washing or looking after the children for a couple of hours. This encouragement and help made a big difference to us all, especially me.

The writing process has been very therapeutic for me. It provides me with a creative outlet which I have total control over. I can write what I want, when I want. It has helped me to get the thoughts out of my head and clarify my emotions. Clarification has then allowed me to analyse my emotions and consider what actions might be required to improve my mental health. A study by Baikie & Wilhelm found that,

> *Writing about traumatic, stressful or emotional events has been found to result in improvements in both physical and psychological health in non-clinical and clinical populations. In the expressive writing paradigm, participants are asked to write about such events for 15-20 minutes on 3-5 occasions. Those who do so generally have significantly better physical and psychological outcomes compared with those who write about neutral topics.* [23]

The feedback I received from family and friends about my blog was very encouraging. Their responses gave me the confidence to further explore this writing gift that had been locked away during ten years of bearing and raising young children. It was one of the catalysts for compiling my blog posts into this book, which I pray will be a blessing in many ways to all who read it.

Chapter 13

School and Another MRI

BLOG POSTS – 31ST JAN TO 15TH FEB 2013

BLOG POST ON 31ST JANUARY 2013

Well, what an emotional roller coaster we have been on in the last forty-eight hours. This scripture certainly sums it up for me.

> *But you, O LORD, are a shield for me, My glory, and the One who lifts my head. I cried to the LORD with my voice, And He heard me from His holy hill. Selah. I lay down and slept; I awoke, for the LORD sustained me. (Psalm 3:2-5 NKJV)*

Tuesday 29th January, 10am we arrived at the hospital for the day-long process of having the MRI. Children under the age of seven requiring an MRI have a general anaesthetic to ensure they are completely still. So Victoria has to fast from 6am that day until after the scan which normally is mid-afternoon.

Thankfully Victoria does not have to stay on the ward while waiting for the MRI. We visited the Starlight Express room, where Victoria and Alexandra treated everyone to a song and dance concert. They did some painting on paper covered balloons, Granny Bett's favourite craft, not. Then Alexandra had her first experience with an electronic game gadget.

While we were in the Starlight Express Room I had the opportunity to chat with some other mums with children with cancer: One Mum, whose daughter had Leukaemia, was very apprehensive about her returning to school the next day, after three terms of absence; Another mum, whose daughter, only about two and a half years old had had a tumour on her shoulder and two in her lungs. She had finished her treatment and was having scans to see if there had been any growth. I salute and honour these mums who have given everything for their children and were still smiling and laughing. It is a very tough journey. Everyone has a story to tell.

After coming out of recovery, Victoria couldn't wait to have a butter sandwich. At 4.45pm we left the hospital, and now wait for the results next week.

All was looking good for Victoria's first day of Kindergarten, Wednesday 29th January, until she woke up. Victoria was complaining of a headache, probably caused by falling

SCHOOL AND ANOTHER MRI

out of bed for the first time ever that previous night. Due to her treatment we are unable to give her pain relief unless advised by the doctor.

As I checked the back of her head, I saw a red patch in amongst her hair. Hair, which is growing back, praise God for that.

The red patch sent me into a panic, as only 2 weeks ago the doctor was telling me to be very careful that Victoria didn't bump her head due to low platelet levels. Even riding a bike was a no-no.

Victoria seemed to be ok when she was distracted, so I decided that she could at least go to kindergarten for a couple of hours and then I would take her up to the hospital to get checked out.

I can't express the disappointment that was in my heart. All had been so perfect for a great start to kindergarten. Who would have thought that she would fall out of bed!

However, I had to gather myself together rather quickly to give Victoria the encouragement she needed for a great first morning. Victoria's official start time on the first day was 8.45am. We were so proud of her.

VICTORIA GRACE

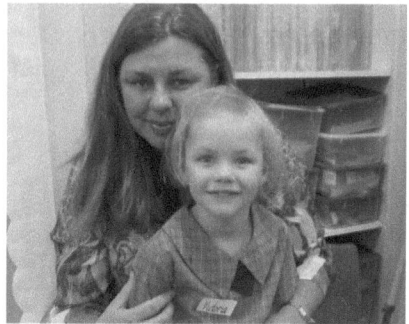

Wendy and Victoria on first day of Kindergarten at Belmont Christian College

Due to the bump on her head, I had planned to pick Victoria up at midday. But by 11am the school had contacted me as she was very distraught about her head. The beautiful teachers, including her Prep teacher from last year had tried to console her, but to no avail. Charlotte had given Victoria all her morning tea and lunch to help her feel better too.

The fears flowed as I drove back to school with a heavy heart. Praise God for the Hillsong worship song, Beneath the waters, I am sure all of Belmont could hear me singing it, well really yelling.

So off to the John Hunter Hospital we went. It was very quiet in the Paediatric Oncology Day Unit, so Victoria could be seen immediately.

After a thorough examination, we were given assurance that the red spot on her head was just the start of a bruise, and then some Panadol was administered. Back to school she went. All was good. Victoria was able to enjoy the

SCHOOL AND ANOTHER MRI

last hour of school with her friends, and at dinner that night couldn't wait to tell us all about school. There was no mention of the hospital visit.

As for me, Ken and my mum, we were utterly emotionally exhausted by the day's events. I am so grateful to God for providing me with the scripture Psalm 3:3-5 in the morning before these events took place, especially verse 5,

> *I lay down and slept;*
> *I awoke, for the Lord sustained me.*
> (Psalm 3:5 NKJV)

Indeed He does sustain me and He knows what we need before we know ourselves.

Now we have the challenge of remaining in peace until we get the MRI results next Wednesday. Without God we would most certainly be a fumbling mess for the entire wait. At least with God, we have His strength to help us face each day and live with hope.

PRAYER POINTS

- ❤ Victoria can complete this first week of kindergarten without any more hospital visits

- ❤ We can remain in God's peace as we wait for the results

♥ For His peace and love to reign in the hearts of other families who are on this similar journey

Many many thanks again for all your prayers and support. Every day we rely more and more on our Heavenly Father to sustain us.

A friend recently told us there was a photo of Victoria and another little boy in the January edition of the Hunter New England Health Matters Magazine, HNE Matters. The story was about the Christmas activities at the John Hunter Hospital. I normally get a copy of this publication when we are at the hospital, and find it fascinating to read about all the great initiatives that are being undertaken here in the Hunter, in all aspects of healthcare. It has opened my eyes to yet another new group of amazing, intelligent and caring people.

> *When Victoria started school I put a few notes together for her teacher regarding Victoria's physical and emotional needs, along with strategies we use to help her when problems arise. Over the years this has grown into a booklet.*

> Appendix H has a contents outline and examples of the information in the booklet.
>
> My prayer is that this will be useful for other families in this situation.

BLOG POST ON 6TH FEBRUARY 2013

Well, today has been one of those days when I just wanted to scream, why can't life be easy and simple?????

The scripture God gave me this morning as I was doing my devotions was from 2 Timothy 1:7,

> *For God did not give us a spirit of timidity (of cowardice, or craven and cringing and fawning fear), but [He has given us a spirit] of power and of love and of calm and of well-balanced mind and discipline and self-control.* (2 Timothy 1:7)

Well, I will say upfront, I certainly needed to call on that spirit of calm, well-balanced mind, discipline and self-control today.

On the way to the appointment with the neurosurgeon to get the results of Victoria's scan my car broke down.

It just stopped in the middle of the traffic. I buried my head in my hands and howled.

Thankfully, and believe me it was difficult to find something to be thankful for, I was only a hundred metres from Ken's office, so he was able to come and rescue me. Ken, with the help of another man, pushed the car to the side of the road. Then I commandeered Ken's car and sped, within the speed limit of course, off to school to pick up Victoria, and then on to the appointment.

Finally we made it to the neurosurgeon's office, 30 minutes late, only to wait another hour before seeing him. The wait actually gave me time to gather myself together Thankfully I had that time, as the scan results were ok, but not what we had hoped and prayed for.

The scans indicate that the tumour is stable. This means the chemotherapy is holding it at its current size, for which are very grateful. This report, of course is better than having the tumour growing. However it does mean that other options will have to be investigated. We will find out more about those options tomorrow when we meet with the oncologist.

We thank God that despite her circumstances Victoria is loving life. She is having a great time at kindergarten, excelling at swimming lessons and is eagerly awaiting starting Girls Brigade next week. Taking the bus to and from school is definitely a highlight in her day.

SCHOOL AND ANOTHER MRI

For those who are interested, and it can make for some scary reading, I came across this very good description of the tumour that is in Victoria's brain on the cancer.net website. It is in the glioma category, and is a low grade pilocytic astrocytoma, located in her brain stem. This website provides a good description of the treatment options for this type of tumour.

> *Note, when we speak about the tumour, we say "the tumour in Victoria's brain", rather than Victoria's tumour, as we do not believe that the tumour belongs to Victoria.*
>
> *It has absolutely no right to be in her brain, in Jesus Name.*

If you do foray into these websites, please keep in mind, that while they describe the situation and options, they of course don't take into account God's sovereignty and His healing power. It is God in whom we choose to put our faith.

BLOG POST ON 10TH FEBRUARY 2013

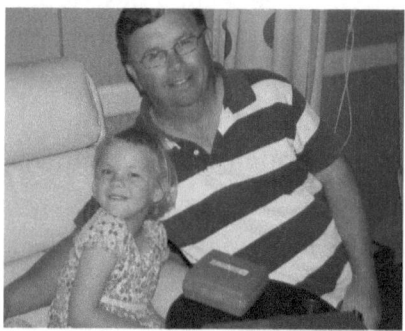

Victoria and Ken in the Paediatric Oncology Day Unit at John Hunter Children's Hospital.

Thank you to everyone who has been praying for our family in the past few days. We have made it through, have regained strength and are ready to face this next week.

How true this scripture is:

> *You, Lord, are forgiving and good, abounding in love to all who call to you. Hear my prayer, LORD; listen to my cry for mercy. When I am in distress, I call to you, because you answer me.* (Psalm 86:5-7 NIV)

Victoria's hair has started to grow back, it is almost an inch long all over. The fact that she didn't go bald was an answer to prayer.

The visit to the oncologist on Thursday confirmed what the neurosurgeon had told us. The tumour is stable.

SCHOOL AND ANOTHER MRI

Chemotherapy will continue until July. Victoria just completed week thirty-two of treatment. Only twenty weeks to go.

In July, the chemotherapy treatment will stop. Victoria will have scans every three months to review what the tumour is doing. If the tumour remains stable and Victoria's health remains good nothing will be done. If the tumour grows again, another twelve month course of chemotherapy will be considered. The goal of the chemotherapy is to prevent or delay radiation therapy. Our prayer is that Victoria will remain well and the chemotherapy will prevent radiation. Surgery is no longer an option, the risks outweigh the benefits.

As for my car, we got it back from the repair shop yesterday, thanks to a wonderful mechanic who worked all day Saturday for us. And thanks to the generosity of a wonderful friend, we had the finance to pay for it. God definitely does listen to our cries for mercy and answers them.

Saturday afternoon we had a very early celebration for my mum's 70th birthday. Mum has been here from New Zealand for the past two and a half weeks. She has been an amazing support, sticking with us as we ride the ups and downs of this journey, not shrinking back when the going gets tough. It was fantastic to relax and have some fun after two weeks of difficult trials. Yes, in the midst of the past two weeks, Ken's office flooded twice!

On a completely different note, Camp Quality asked us to attend a camp this weekend as a 'mentor family' to families who have just received a diagnosis in the past twelve months. It is an honour to be asked, and overwhelming at the same time, as we are still in the midst of our journey. But then, so is God. He hears us, listens to us and answers us - these past two weeks have been testimony to that truth.

PRAYER POINTS

- ♥ We will continue to fix our eyes on Jesus, despite the trials that come our way

- ♥ Victoria will remain well as she mixes with children at school

- ♥ Our family will be effective mentors at the Camp Quality new families camp

Thank you so much again for your prayers, please do not underestimate their power. Thank you, too, for the practical support and encouraging emails. We need it all.

BLOG POST ON 15TH FEBRUARY 2013

This week Victoria went to the John Hunter Hospital for chemotherapy on Wednesday, so Alexandra was able to accompany us. What a great time she had on an ergonomic chair, with a seat rather like a saddle.

SCHOOL AND ANOTHER MRI

Alexandra even thought it might make a good motorbike seat, with the bed-end being the handlebars.

The nurses in the day unit were delighted to see the girls' smiling faces and loved hearing the songs that Victoria had learnt at Prep, including the one about Mrs Brown who went to town with her underpants down. Victoria was pleased to have Alexandra with us for the day.

It seems that Wednesday's are a quieter day in the Paediatric Oncology Day Unit, so rather than waiting for the blood results in the treatment room, we were able to wait in the reception area.

The girls watched a movie and then did some colouring and play at the little table. We had to wait about two and a half hours for the blood results, as when Victoria's neutrophils are reported as low, additional checks need to be done. They confirmed that her neutrophil count was only 0.3 so she was unable to have chemotherapy this week.

We are thankful to God that Victoria has remained well these past two days and we are on track to attend the Camp Quality family camp this week. We are all looking forward to a welcome break away from home, even though the camp will have its own emotional challenges. I always cry when we arrive at any of these events, overcome with people's generosity and kind hearts, and very mindful of the reason why we are attending the event.

PRAYER POINTS

♥ That every member of our family will be a blessing to at least one other person at the camp

♥ That all the camp attendees will remain well and safe during the weekend

As we have come through the trials of the past two weeks, I will continue to claim this scripture over our lives, Psalm 23:1-3

> *The LORD is my shepherd, I shall not want. He makes me to lie down in green pastures; He leads me beside the still waters. He restores my soul; He leads me in paths of righteousness for His name's sake.* (Psalm 23:1-3 NKJV)

Thank you again for your prayers and continued practical support of our family.

SCHOOL AND ANOTHER MRI

REFLECTION – FATHERS

It is easy to become a father, but very difficult to be a father. [25]

What a huge responsibility it is to be a father. Obviously I am not one, so I cannot fully understand all that it entails. But I have made some observations over the years.

Two days after we began to understand the magnitude of what Victoria was facing, my father flew over from New Zealand. I remember when he arrived, mid-afternoon on Saturday. We were all at home, Victoria having been discharged for the seven days prior to her operation. The children were swimming in the pool, enjoying a beautiful January summer's day.

My father is not a man of fanfare. He is a quiet, deep-thinking man, for whom expressing emotion does not come easily. On that afternoon, it didn't matter that he didn't have much to say. He was here with us and that was more than enough.

On previous visits, my dad's time had normally been spent working through a list of home maintenance jobs. Mum and I usually put the list together. We greatly appreciate all the handiwork he has done around our home.

However, on this trip, there was no list. The goings on for each day were unknown. The outcome of each day was unknown. I cannot begin to imagine how this time of uncertainty was for my father.

As with my mum and sister, there were times of emotional distance between us resulting from words spoken in moments of high stress. It was a period of stretching and growing our relationship. Ultimately these challenges have led to a greater level of love and respect.

There is a silent strength about my father that I appreciate even more now, after all we have been through with Victoria. Karen Boyer's poem expresses this well.

> *SILENT STRONG DAD*
> *by Karen K. Boyer* [26]
>
> *He never looks for praises*
> *He's never one to boast*
> *He just goes on quietly working*
> *For those he loves the most*
> *His dreams are seldom spoken*
> *His wants are very few*
> *And most of the time his worries*
> *Will go unspoken too*
> *He's there ... A firm foundation*
> *Through all our storms of life*
> *A sturdy hand to hold to*
> *In times of stress and strife*
> *A true friend we can turn to*
> *When times are good or bad*

SCHOOL AND ANOTHER MRI

One of our greatest blessings,
The man that we call Dad.

Neither do I really know how it was for Ken, as Victoria's father, when she was diagnosed. He was inter-state so not able to be at the hospital and I imagine he was feeling helpless. I do know he spent a lot of that night talking to his mother on the phone.

I also know that he spent a lot of time crying out to God, knowing there was nothing he himself could do to fix the situation. This wasn't like a business problem, where Ken could draw on his skills, experience and perseverance to change things. None of those attributes would help him help Victoria. His only option was to trust God, that He would provide the right people to help our daughter. Not an easy thing to do, especially when you are used to solving problems. Thankfully, by the grace of God, we were able to come together and remind each other that we had to keep on looking to our Heavenly Father, trusting that He had a plan for us and it was good.

When Victoria was discharged from hospital following brain surgery, Ken's focus needed to return fully to our business. It became my responsibility then to take Victoria to all the physical therapy appointments, chemotherapy treatments and scans. Ken's involvement was reduced to attending the oncologist appointments to get the MRI results.

As time went on, Victoria's weekly chemotherapy regime started to take a toll on me. We noticed a pattern had developed with the emergency hospital visits. These usually occurred in third week of the chemotherapy cycle, when Victoria would often become febrile. After some discussion, we adjusted our emergency plan. If the high temperatures occurred on the Friday or Saturday, Ken would take Victoria to hospital for the first night. We would swap over the following morning. This change to our contingency plans gave me the opportunity to organise the other children at home and to reduce the amount of time I was away from them.

It also gave Ken a way to be more involved with Victoria's care, adding a new dimension for Victoria in the hospital, because as we know, Daddy does things differently to Mummy. Victoria often recalls with a laugh, when she went to hospital with Daddy and asked him for a chocolate bar. Daddy dutifully went and bought a chocolate bar. But rather than returning with a small 50gm block of chocolate, he had a 250gm block, much to Victoria's delight - not that she probably felt like eating it.

Ken's father too has been a practical support to our family. When Ken's parents looked after Alexandra at home in the early days of chemotherapy treatment, Ken's Dad would do all our ironing. With six people in the family, there was always a lot of it to be done. It was a bonus to come home from hospital and find all the ironing completed.

SCHOOL AND ANOTHER MRI

These three fathers, my dad, Ken, and his father, have all made the choice to stick with their family, love and support them and not give up. In their own ways they have modelled aspects of what being a loving father is. Our children and I are so blessed to have them in our lives, choosing to love us.

I know that not everyone has earthly fathers like these. But even these three fathers are not perfect, and that is where our Heavenly Father comes in. He fills the gaps of our imperfect earthly fathers. He fills the gap left by absent fathers, or those who are now in heaven. Our Heavenly Father is always there, responding immediately with love and grace.

> *See what great love the Father has lavished on us, that we should be called children of God! And that is what we are!* (1 John 3:1 NIV)

Chapter 14

Normal Life

BLOG POSTS – 19TH FEB TO 29TH MAR 2013

BLOG POST ON 19TH FEBRUARY 2013

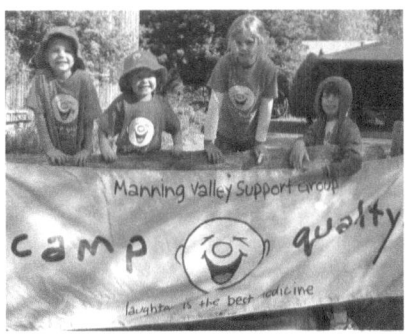

Victoria, Alexandra, Charlotte and Marshall at Riverwood Downs, Barrington Tops, NSW.

> *Thank [God] in everything [no matter what the circumstances may be, be thankful and give thanks] for this is the will of God for you [who are] in Christ Jesus [the Revealer and Mediator of that will].*
> (1 Thessalonians 5:18)

We do have so much to be thankful for, despite all the things that are thrown at us as a family, we continue to experience God's blessing and favour on all our lives.

We attended a Camp Quality family camp at Riverwood Downs at the foothills of Barrington Tops, a world heritage wilderness. We were spoilt in 4.5 star resort rooms set amidst beautiful gardens.

We all enjoyed the many activities made available for us, including canoeing on the river. Ken, Victoria and Alexandra easily won the up-stream race. Marshall, Charlotte and I found it difficult to go in a straight line, and constantly went from one side of the river to the other. This could possibly have been due to the lack of co-ordination between our 3 paddles. Tubing down the river was another activity enjoyed by Ken, Marshall, Charlotte and me.

On the Saturday afternoon two oncology social workers from Redkite came down from Brisbane to run a parents' group. The purpose of the group was to provide a relaxed, informal get-together where we could chat with other parents about the impact of childhood cancer on you and your family. Both Ken and I found the group very beneficial, as although each family's experience is unique there are many commonalities in terms of the trauma experienced at the time of diagnosis and coping mechanisms throughout the journey. While we attended the parent group the children were busy in the craft room.

After the parent group it was time for some relaxation in the pool. Riverwood Downs is just magnificent, and with the recent rain it was all so green.

Sunday morning we had the opportunity to go horse-riding. The children were led around the paddock on various horses. After they had finished their rides, they were taken back to the camp and looked after by the Camp Quality volunteers. The parents were then invited to ride the horses on a trail over the paddocks, up hills and through the trees. It was great fun. No one fell off.

All in all we had a fantastic weekend away. It was great to get outdoors and marvel at God's beautiful world. It was equally good to have some laughs as a family.

PRAYER POINTS

- Victoria is well enough to have chemotherapy this week

- Strength and energy for Ken and I as we face the challenges this circumstance brings

Thank you again for your prayers and practical support. We are forever grateful.

BLOG POST ON 21ST FEBRUARY 2013

Victoria had enough neutrophils to have chemo yesterday. Praise God.

After discussing schooling impacts with Victoria's teacher I decided to change her treatment day to Wednesday, mid-morning, with the approval of the doctors of course. This means she can go to school and learn the phonogram for the day, and then go to hospital and do her homework. Well, that is the theory anyway.

This change in routine also means that Alexandra will be joining us each Wednesday. She is now old enough to sit for the required length of time. If necessary we can go for a walk with the buzzer while waiting for the blood test results to come back, and the receptionist will buzz us when the doctor needs us to return. We normally have to wait 45 minutes to an hour for the blood to be analysed.

This afternoon I have had an interesting telephone conversation with Victoria's Occupational Therapist. We were discussing Victoria's eyesight and she suggested I try the following, to understand better what Victoria can and can't see. Why not give it a go....

1. Put on a pair of glasses

2. On the left lense, put a yellow sticky note covering from the centre of the lense to the outside of your face

3. On the right lense, put a yellow sticky note covering from the centre of the lens to your nose

Now you have the exact same vision as Victoria. And we have a better understanding of why Victoria tilts her head to the right when she is writing. And so the learning goes on.

Victoria continues to love school and learning the phonograms. Tomorrow she starts circuit training for sport which will be a bit tricky for her and the school athletics carnival is in two weeks.

Please pray that Victoria will not lose confidence and will not stop trying to participate in these physically challenging activities. We believe she will indeed be victorious in all areas of her life and that she will know the peace of her Heavenly Father.

> *When I said, "My foot is slipping", your unfailing love, LORD supported me. When anxiety was great within me, your consolation brought me joy. (Psalm 94:18-19 NIV)*

BLOG POST ON 27TH FEBRUARY 2013

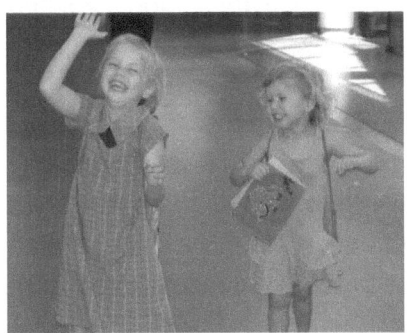

Victoria and Alexandra walking down the main corridor at John Hunter Hospital

VICTORIA GRACE

All went well at treatment yesterday. Looking at this picture, who would have thought that Victoria had just been sitting in the treatment room for the past four hours.

Having Alexandra with us at the hospital now is such a blessing. She watches everything with interest and is so proud of her sibling bravery beads. The other night at "show and tell" at dinner, she showed us all every one. Normally siblings get one bead per visit, however this week Alexandra got five.

The nurses also gave the girls some bags and craft things to take home. They very proudly wore them out of the hospital.

Next Wednesday is an off week, which is great as Victoria can attend the school athletics carnival.

Thank you to everyone who prayed for Victoria's challenge of the circuit at school last week. Being the determined girl that she is, she gave every activity station a go, and most she could do in some way.

I don't often say this or in fact even think it, but today I am just going to put it out there - it is really hard being a family who has a child with cancer. At times the stress on family members is immense. Here is a snippet of an exchange that took place between some of our children last week.

NORMAL LIFE

Child A - I don't want to help *** anymore. Why does she need help anyway?

Child B - Because she has cancer

Child C - Why do I have to be the only one in the family who has cancer?

Obviously this type of conversation doesn't go on every day, or even every week or month. But there are days when it really does get all too much for some of us. Thankfully we have never all felt this way on the same day, so at least one person in the family can stand strong and help the rest of us lift our heads and come back to a place of love and grace.

Victoria has just completed week thirty-four of treatment. She has about four months to go. The next scan is April 16th. This journey has been, and is long. As a mum the challenge to be emotionally and spiritually strong can sometimes be very overwhelming. My gracious Heavenly Father reminded me this morning of Isaiah 40:29-31, particularly verse 31,

> *But those who hope in the LORD will renew their strength. They will soar on wings like eagles; they will run and not grow weary, they will walk and not be faint.* (Isaiah 40:31 NIV)

This truth brings great peace to my heart and a supernatural energy to continue through the day. My mind is now often jumping ahead to what happens after July. It is with every ounce of mental strength I can muster that I bring my mind back to focus only on today. I remind myself of this scripture God gave me back in June 2010 when we were facing other trials, and as with His word, how relevant it is still for me today ...

> *But me, I'm not giving up, I'm sticking around to see what God will do. I'm waiting for God to make things right. I'm counting on God to listen to me.* (Micah 7:7 The Message)

PRAYER POINTS

- ♥ Victoria will continue to have minimal side effects from the chemotherapy

- ♥ Each member of our family will continue to seek God for strength and learn more about how to show His love and compassion to each other

- ♥ Our family will continue to stand strong together and be a light for Jesus

Thank you too for sticking with us.

NORMAL LIFE

BLOG POST ON 7TH MARCH 2013

My word for this week is 'grace'. And the scripture, a favourite,

> But He said to me, My grace (my favour and loving-kindness and mercy) is enough for you [sufficient against any danger and enables you to bear the trouble manfully]; for My strength and power are made perfect (fulfilled and completed) and show themselves most effective in [your] weakness. Therefore I will all the more gladly glory in my weakness and infirmities, that the strength and power of Christ (the Messiah) may rest (yes, may pitch a tent over and dwell) upon me!
> (2 Corinthians 12:9)

God has lovingly poured out his grace on me this past week. It has been filled with many tears. I have gone through another period of grieving the expectations of how our family would be at this time and what we would be doing. Tuesday night this week was the worst, in fact as I was crying myself to sleep I cried out to God, "Enough! Tomorrow is the school athletics carnival and I know Victoria won't be able to do some of the activities, but please let her enjoy the day, and please help me to get through the day without any tears."

In His graciousness, we had the best day at the carnival. Victoria participated in what she could, and when she couldn't her loving gracious teacher found an alternative way for her to be involved. Victoria herself showed strength and grace by cheering on her friends in the 100m race, as she watched from the side lines.

Another act of God's grace that I have reflected on this morning, was Charlotte's performance at the carnival. To our surprise she placed in the 400m and 800m race. I felt God say to me this morning, she has the determination and character to go the distance, to run the race of life and run it well. What peace that brought to my heart. His grace really is sufficient for us all.

As for my tears, there was only one moment in the day when I felt the tears well up, while talking to one of the beautiful caring school mums. And that was it. I was so thankful that I could maintain a smile for the entire day.

Last Thursday we attended the VIP night at the Newcastle Show. The children had a great time on the rides. Marshall enjoyed the more daring rides, while the girls enjoyed honing their driving skills. Although, I am not sure if Alexandra was totally confident in Charlotte's driving ability.

What a difference it makes not having to go up to the hospital for treatment this week. We have almost had a doctor/medical visit free week, but not quite.

Victoria's legs have been troubling her, so we did go to see the physiotherapist on Tuesday. Victoria's right leg is still tighter than her left leg, although less tight than in January, Praise God. The tightness is making walking difficult. She has been unable to wear the right leg night boot due to this stiffness. The physiotherapist made a new night boot for her right leg with less of a stretch than the previous one. Victoria has worn the boot successfully for two nights now.

I feel for her as I see her wriggling in bed with both boots on, trying to get comfortable. And I wonder, how much more will she have to endure?

PRAYER POINTS

- ♥ Thank you to God for his amazing grace

- ♥ Please pray that Victoria's leg muscles will continue to stretch and that she will walk using her entire right foot, not just on tippee toes

For anyone who is interested, I have been re-reading a little book, only thirty-seven pages, called Good Grief [27] by Granger E. Westberg. I have found it explains the stages of grief very simply. And if you are grieving something, it helps you to know that what you are feeling at a particular point in time is normal.

BLOG POST ON 16TH MARCH 2013

God's blessing and favour is on us despite our

circumstances. We have just had four nights away courtesy of the Starlight Children's foundation and NRMA Ocean Beach Holiday Park. These organisations really understand the value of families "getting away" just to be a family having fun.

It was an absolute joy to have so much time just to 'be' with our children and marvel at how resilient they are. And how loving and caring they can be towards each other most of the time! Riding in the buggies was a display of this, as Marshall drove Victoria and Charlotte drove Alexandra.

Victoria and Alexandra thought that they would have a go together. They didn't get to go anywhere, their legs weren't quite long enough.

As the four of them road down the path together, I wanted to yell out, "God is good, these children are a testimony of His goodness."

This morning God gave me this scripture in relation to our children,

> *God is with them, and they're with him, shouting praises to their King. God brought them out of Egypt rampaging like a wild ox.* (Numbers 23:21-22 The Message)

I am standing on that verse.

NORMAL LIFE

On Wednesday of course Victoria had chemotherapy back at the John Hunter Hospital. As we drove there from the Central Coast, it made me think about those families who have to drive that distance or further each week once or twice for treatment. I again thanked God that we were living in close proximity to a hospital able to provide the treatment Victoria needed when she was first diagnosed.

It was a very quiet day in the Paediatric Oncology Day Unit; we were the only ones there. The children were able to make themselves at home. Victoria was well enough to have chemotherapy this week. The doctors were concerned about an infection in her arm. Thankfully after prayer and antibiotics, when we returned to the hospital for a check-up yesterday, the infection appeared to be going.

Changing treatment day to Wednesday has many advantages, including easier access to the psychologist assigned to the Paediatric Oncology Department. The topic of conversation this week was Victoria's adjustment to moving from the safe environments of home, hospital and prep school into the big wide world of school.

An insight into how Victoria currently views herself came from this conversation at the camp ground. We were sitting next to a father and his son. We were putting on Victoria's socks, splint and shoes, when Victoria volunteered this information to the father, "This is my splint. It helps me walk better. I feel weird because I have a splint." Thankfully the gracious father responded by saying, "It is just part of you."

Please pray for us as we help Victoria to understand that she is not weird, she is just different and that is ok. And more importantly that she will believe her Heavenly Father says she is "wonderfully and fearfully made". Psalm 139:14

Once again I thank God for this time away, as these sorts of conversations and valuable insights don't happen in the hub-bub of normal life and can easily be missed in the 'circus' that is the Robinson household.

The strength in her legs continues to increase as she runs and jumps effortlessly up and down the jumping pillow. Freedom! This is a testimony of the healing that is happening in Victoria's body.

PRAYER POINTS

- ♥ Victoria will know in her heart that she is fearfully and wonderfully made

- ♥ The infection will continue to disappear

- ♥ Peace to reign in our hearts as the next scan draws closer on the 16th April

NORMAL LIFE

BLOG POST ON 21ST MARCH 2013

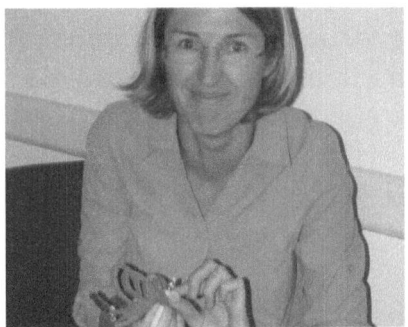

My sister doing craft in the Paediatric Oncology Day Unit, John Hunter Children's Hospital.

Victoria was well enough to have chemo yesterday, despite her neutrophils being on the low side. Praise God. The infection in her arm has almost cleared up. Again we are thankful that it did not spread.

We were able to visit the Starlight Express room while waiting for the blood results. One of the Captain's was doing face painting. Alexandra gladly put her hand up.

The Starlight Express room craft for the morning involved pipe cleaners, beads and calico bags. For the super-crafty you could have a go at poking the pipe cleaners through the calico and adding beads to make beautiful patterns. We chose to stick with slightly simpler things. My sister, visiting from New Zealand made some butterflies and spiders. I helped Victoria make a necklace.

Emotionally this week everyone is travelling pretty well. Although dolly came with us to the hospital this trip, as she had the vomits during the night. Thank you for your prayer covering. Last week while we were away I listened to a podcast from a wonderful friend from Sydney. It helped me to examine my thoughts and get them lined up with God's truth.

As we draw closer to another scan, God's word continues to be a marvellous comfort.

> *Asa cried to the Lord his God, O Lord, there is none besides You to help, and it makes no difference to You whether the one You help is mighty or powerless. Help us, O Lord our God! For we rely on You and we go against this multitude in Your name. O Lord, You are our God; let no man prevail against you.* (2 Chronicles 14:11)

Many, many thanks again for the continued prayer and practical support. You are a blessing, in Jesus' Name.

BLOG POST ON 29TH MARCH 2013

This past week has been a time of reflection. Prior to Victoria's diagnosis I didn't think much about Heaven. I lived gladly with the knowledge that accepting Jesus as my Lord and Saviour meant, among other things, I had the assurance that Heaven is where I will spend eternity.

Since Victoria's diagnosis, at various times, thoughts of

NORMAL LIFE

Heaven have been at the forefront of my mind. It is not that I don't believe that God can perform miracles, I do believe that. But I also know that God is sovereign.

I don't want our children to fear death. I want them to know that Heaven is a beautiful place where everything is perfect. To help them with that understanding, I have bought the book Heaven is for real for kids [28] and have read it with our eldest child. He has an enquiring mind and is now listening to the audio book of the full version.

One of the things we know for sure about our life as a Christian is that Heaven is our destination at some point in time. I don't want our children to be afraid of that truth.

Victoria was able to have chemotherapy this week. No infections, all good. We had a session with the occupational therapist, who has given us exercises to start training Victoria to scan to the left when moving around. Next week is a week off treatment.

On a completely different note, for anyone who enjoys contemporary worship, here is a song that for me is like stepping into a refreshing shower, You Revive Me by Christy Nockels. I can highly recommend sitting quietly and letting the words flow over you, into your heart. Let Jesus revive you this Easter weekend.

VICTORIA GRACE

REFLECTION – SIBLINGS ARE A BLESSING

Often we hear about fights between siblings, a complete lack of respect and appreciation. I pray that this reflection on the positive aspects of siblings is a blessing to you, and where there is friction, I pray that God will bring restoration.

My only sister, Allison, has been a blessing to us throughout this journey, especially in the first few weeks. I remember when I told her the news of Victoria's diagnosis. She was on holiday in Australia with her husband and daughter. It was the morning after Victoria had had the CT scan, when Allison phoned, 'Hi, how is everything going?'

Still in shock over Victoria's diagnosis, my reply was feeble, 'We are at the hospital. There is a mass in Victoria's brain.'

There was a scream on the other end of the phone. Then without any hesitation, Allison said, 'We'll come straight away.'

That response sums up my sister. Throughout this journey she has always been there when I have needed her, with either practical or emotional support. I can still picture Allison running down the hospital corridor pushing her daughter in the stroller. And the sense of relief I had when I saw her, the same feeling I had when my mum arrived at the hospital an hour or so earlier. I don't know how we would have made it through the next two weeks without them. It certainly made things easier, both at home and at hospital.

But as with any high stress situation, there were moments during these three years when our relationship was tested. For my sister and me, these resulted from words spoken in extremely traumatic situations, lack of communication or differing expectations. However, with time, grace and forgiveness, eventually there has always been restoration. It is as though we have an unspoken understanding that the sister bond is greater than any of these moments, and we need to do whatever is necessary to prevent our connection being permanently broken. As hard as these moments were, I feel that they were 'moments of growth', ultimately resulting in a more authentic and emotionally healthy sister relationship.

Ken's only sister, Michelle, has also been a blessing during this journey. She provided emotional support to Ken's parents as they navigated this journey as grandparents.

This story involves other sibling relationships, the ones between Victoria and her siblings. Marshall, Charlotte and Alexandra have been an indescribable blessing to Victoria. They were all so young when she was diagnosed; Marshall aged seven, Charlotte five, and Alexandra only one year old. They have been closely involved with this whole journey, whether it was hanging out at the hospital in the days before Victoria's brain surgery, or attending physiotherapy and occupational therapy appointments, or coming to the chemotherapy treatments. Each of them, in their own way, has supported her. Marshall quietly took on the protective big brother role at such a young age. Charlotte, always thinking of ways to help her sister, bringing toys and food up to the hospital, all while trying to work out how to handle her own emotions. Alexandra, not really old enough to understand what was going on, probably just thought hospital was her second home and it was normal to be there every couple of days.

I asked Victoria how her siblings have helped her, especially when she was in hospital. Here is what she had to say.

> 'Marshall always calms me down in the night, giving me a hug. He helps me to walk around and do stuff I can't do. And he encourages me to be brave and stay strong.'
>
> Charlotte is encouraging to me and helps me with my goals with maths, spelling, reading and computers. She read books to me in hospital when I was sad.'
>
> Alexandra makes me laugh. She cuddles me when I am sad. In hospital she would sit with me and watch TV with me and make funny jokes with me.'

Marshall, Charlotte and Alexandra have also been a blessing in relation to the physical challenges Victoria experiences with hemiplegia. Being one of four children,

NORMAL LIFE

Victoria always wants to keep up with the others, even when her body won't fully allow her to. For example, if they are running around playing 'tips', then Victoria too is running around playing tips. If they are diving into the pool, racing to the other end, then Victoria is right there in the mix. How different this scenario would have been if she'd not had siblings. That natural level of physical activity just wouldn't have happened. We would have witnessed a lot of muscle wastage and reduced functionality in what Victoria could do.

We are so proud of how our other children have supported Victoria, but recognise that they too needed support. As the Redkite [29] organisation explains,

> *Having a brother or sister with cancer changes a child's life a great deal. It is natural and unavoidable that your child with cancer will receive more of your time and attention but it is also natural for your other children to react to this change in your relationship. Common reactions are:*
>
> - *Difficulty in understanding and accepting the extra attention that their sick brother or sister is receiving*
>
> - *Worrying about who will look after them when you are unavailable because of treatment and hospital visits*

- *Feeling scared and sorry for their sick brother or sister*

- *Feeling angry about all of the changes, and sometimes with their sick brother or sister*

- *Feeling guilty and believing they may have somehow caused the cancer*

- *Behavioural changes such as headaches, problems at school, and attention seeking can be common*

Over the years we have seen each of these reactions in our children at different times. We know that our children have their own ways of processing and expressing their feelings. As you have read in this book, we have made use of many of the support services available to families of children with cancer, to ensure that we all come out of this journey as emotionally healthy as possible. We are grateful for all these organisations, including the ones who offer support for the whole family, like Camp Quality and the Starlight Children's Foundation.

We have always worked towards educating the children, age appropriately, about what is happening in Victoria's body. The Medikidz graphic novels were one series of books that Marshall related well to. The three Medikidz books that were particularly relevant to our circumstance were Brain Tumours; Stroke and Acquired Brain Injury.

NORMAL LIFE

When talking about these medical conditions, we always included some discussion about Jesus and His healing power, reminding the children that we have faith that complete healing will manifest in Victoria's body. But at the same time we acknowledge that right now Victoria has to live with these conditions which may give her extra physical pain and tiredness, and mental fatigue. And it is important that we as a family are aware of these impacts and demonstrate grace towards her.

Redkite [30] also provides some suggestions for how to help the siblings of your unwell child.

- *Talk with them about how they feel*

- *Talk with them about the cancer, the treatment, and care.*

- *Spend time with them*

- *Have clear plans about who will be looking after them and let them know about those plans*

- *Encourage them to take part in outside activities*

- *Involve them in their brother's or sister's treatment but without making unreasonable demands*

- *Talk with them about questions their schoolmates and friends may ask*

- *Know who their favourite family members, friends and other trusted adults are and keep those people informed. Organise for your children to spend time with them when possible*

- *Explain why they need to be taken care of by other family members and friends while your sick child undergoes treatment*

We have taken on board all these suggestions during this journey and found that they have been a great guide in helping us support our children. Just as we have continually sought to frame everything that goes on in our lives as a picture of God's grace. It has been important for us that all our children understand that God isn't the source of bad things that happen to our family. However, He does equip us with all we need to get through these difficult circumstances. God is developing our character every step of the way so that we can go on to do all that He has called us to do. We have done our best to teach our children to stick with God no matter what.

> 'For this very reason, make every effort to add to your faith goodness, and to goodness, knowledge; and to knowledge, self-control; and to self-control, perseverance; and to perseverance, godliness; and to godliness, mutual affection;

and to mutual affection, love. For if you possess these qualities in increasing measure, they will keep you from being ineffective and unproductive in your knowledge of our Lord Jesus Christ. (2 Peter 1:3-8 NIV)

Sibling relationships can be challenging. As I said at the beginning of this reflection, I pray that where there is friction in a sibling relationship, God will bring humility, forgiveness and complete restoration. Siblings are a blessing.

Chapter 15

Living From Scan to Scan

BLOG POSTS – 9TH APR TO 21ST MAY 2013

BLOG POST ON 9TH APRIL 2013

Victoria enjoyed a great morning at school last week at the Kings and Queens day. Although with her home-made crown Marshall wondered if she was going to audition for the role of Pope.

Unfortunately, she couldn't get to stay the whole day at school as she had an infection on her leg which needed hospital attention, so we didn't get to have a hospital-free week. One bonus during the hospital visit, was that Victoria got the opportunity to meet a special dog that was brought into hospital to add some joy to the children's day.

On Friday at school she gave a presentation to her class, taking them on a journey into her other world, the hospital. Victoria told them about her Wednesday hospital activities. She also explained to her class how they could help her out physically at school. I was so proud of Victoria, especially when she explained how it was helpful if they walked on her left side so she didn't bump into things, and if they didn't know which her left side was, they just had to look at which leg had the splint on. She is such a brave and courageous child.

'You live from scan to scan.' When Victoria was diagnosed these were some of the first words I heard from a parent of a child living with cancer. At the time I really had no idea what they meant. However after Victoria had had a few scans I understood. When I gained that understanding, I started living from 'scan to scan'.

I would find myself getting more and more anxious as the scan date drew closer, and even more nervous as we waited the week or so after the scan to find out what the results were. Then once we knew the results, I relaxed into normal life for a couple of months, before starting on the anxiety treadmill again. And so the cycle repeated itself every three months for the past two years. This was not an emotionally healthy cycle for me.

Now I find myself with a different understanding, thanks to a scripture I read last week from The Message Bible.

> *'You let the world, which doesn't know the first thing about living, tell you how to live'.*
> (Ephesians 2:1a The Message)

For a few days I meditated on this verse, before I began to fully understand what God was trying to say to me. I had the revelation that God wants me to live each day in His rest, regardless of what is happening on that day, regardless of what is spoken to me that day, and regardless of how I feel on that day. Now that is a big ask given our circumstances, but I fully believe that God can help me get to the point where I can live each day like that, and no longer live 'from scan to scan'. I would appreciate your prayers as I pursue God's perfect rest, peace and joy for every day.

Victoria and Charlotte are off to a Camp Quality camp this weekend, so could you please pray for complete health for both girls in the next few days and during the camp. It is such a wonderful opportunity for them both.

Many thanks for your wonderful on-going support in so many ways.

BLOG POST ON 15TH APRIL 2013

Charlotte and Victoria returned from the Camp Quality Junior Camp at Point Wolstoncroft, Lake Macquarie, late yesterday afternoon. They had an awesome time and were so well looked after by their companions. We are so grateful to Camp Quality and the opportunities and fun they give us all. While the girls were canoeing, disco dancing and doing lots of craft, we were enjoying two days of being a family of four. The house was so quiet and tidy!

The camp was a great way to start the school holidays, and a week full of hospital visits, Tuesday, MRI and physio, Wednesday, OT and Thursday, Chemo and scan results. It is never dull here.

We continue to believe for a good result from the scan. Physically looking at Victoria there is nothing to indicate that there has been any major growth in the tumour.

PRAYER POINTS

- ♥ Victoria will be well enough to have the general anaesthetic tomorrow for the MRI

- ♥ We will remain in God's peace as we wait for the MRI results and hear the results

- ♥ Victoria will continue to strengthen physically

Many thanks again for your continued prayers and support as we continue to choose to trust God with our daughter.

Some food for thought from a book I am reading, Names of God, by Nathan Stone. In fact I have been stuck on this page for a couple of weeks.

> *It is in this connection that another aspect of the name El-Shaddai, as the One who fills and makes fruitful, appears. We have already seen that to experience God's sufficiency one must*

realise one's own insufficiency. To experience God's fullness one must empty self. It is not easy to empty self. It was never easy to do that. The less empty of self we are, the less of blessing God can pour into us; the more of pride and self-sufficiency, the less fruit we can bear. Sometimes chastening can make us realize this. Thus it is that the name Almighty God or El-Shaddai is used in connection with judging, chastening, purging. ..... And as in the case of Naomi, is it not also true of Job that even this 'perfect and upright' man was made more upright or whole through sufferings; that he was purged, through chastening, of some imperfections that hindered his fullest blessing and fruitfulness, that this chastening emptied him so completely of self that he could be 'filled to the measure of all the fullness of God'? (Ephesians 3:19). He understood this in the day when he said: 'Now my eyes have seen you. Therefore I despise myself and repent in dust and ashes" (Job 42:5-6). Then he received power with God to intercede for his friends, and he was filled with double blessings.' [31]

From on-going personal experience, moving from the Super Miss Self-Sufficient I was eighteen years ago, to the person God is continuingly moulding me into today, I totally agree with Stone, that "It is not easy to empty self". However, with everything we have gone through, I would much prefer to be the person I am now, than that person eighteen years ago. Thank you Heavenly Father, Jesus and Holy Spirit.

> *See what [an incredible] quality of love the Father has given (shown, bestowed on) us, that we should [be permitted to] be named and called and counted the children of God! And so we are!* (1 John 3:1)

BLOG POST ON 18TH APRIL 2013

> *How great is our God, sing with me how great is our God!* [32]

The MRI indicated that the tumour has shrunk by 20%.

On Tuesday the physiotherapist advised that the range in Victoria's ankles were back to normal. She will need to continue wearing the night boots, but there will be no need to take steps to get a day splint for her right leg.

Thank you for continuing to uphold Victoria and our family in prayer. Our God is faithful, all the praise and glory to Him.

Due to this great result, the weekly chemotherapy treatment may be extended another three months to October.

Please pray that throughout this time we will continue to

Set our minds and keep them set on what is above (the higher things), not on the things that are on earth. (Colossians 3:2)

And that Victoria will continue to cope so wonderfully with the treatment, in Jesus' name.

What to do now? Lunch and clean out the kitchen cupboards - what else would you do after such fantastic news?

BLOG POST ON 28TH APRIL 2013

We continue to thank God for the news we received last week. Victoria looks and is so well, despite the weekly chemotherapy regime.

This week I wanted to say a big thank you to everyone, especially our extended families who have supported us tremendously since Victoria was first diagnosed in January 2011. Our parents and siblings have given so much to us in many ways. Without them we would be in a very different 'place' than we are today. They have shown us unconditional love and grace as our emotions have roller-coasted. We thank God for the blessing they are to us.

Victoria has once again been given the opportunity to do Hippotherapy at the Riding for the Disabled Centre at Raymond Terrace. She had an assessment there last

Tuesday, and afterwards we had a picnic in the sensory garden. Alexandra enjoyed looking at the tea cups in the garden.

Victoria's attendance at the weekly sessions is contingent on her platelet levels being high enough. This will be determined by the blood tests she has for chemotherapy each week. We pray that she will be able to attend each of the seven sessions.

God has taught me and continues to teach me many things on this journey. One big concept I am only starting to get a handle on is that God really does have it all under control. I say it, I write it, I believe it - sometimes. But sometimes is not enough. I need to believe it all the time.

I am claiming this truth from Genesis 15:1 over our lives,

> *After these things the word of [Jehovah] came unto Abram in a vision, saying, Fear not, Abram: I am thy shield, and thy exceeding great reward.* (Genesis 15:1)

To this end, I have written a chronological list of the promises and scriptures God has given me personally since I became a Christian in 1996, and a list of the significant events where God has been evident in my life. I have pasted this list into the beginning of my journal, so whenever that ugly fear rises up, I will turn to it and remind myself of the promises God has given me, and that God, my shield, is there protecting me and my family.

Now, on a lighter note, a question - what do you do when your child is hungry and thirsty and can't have anything to eat or drink because they are waiting to have a general anaesthetic and MRI?

Answer: give them your camera to play with... all is good, waiting, waiting ... now Mummy's getting tired of waiting ... so she has a nap.

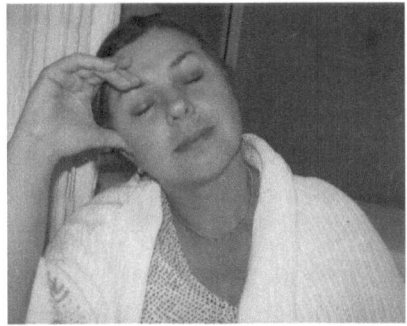

Wendy having a nap while waiting for Victoria's MRI at John Hunter Children's Hospital

I think all that waiting is one of the reasons Mummies get bravery beads too.

BLOG POST ON 7TH MAY 2013

On Sunday Victoria gave me a stark reminder of the thoughts that are in her head and all she has had to cope with, especially during the chemotherapy treatment. She was sitting in the kitchen, holding her dolly Sophie. There was a pile of Sophie's hair on the floor. I inquired as to why she had cut Sophie's hair. The response was, 'Now she looks like me'.

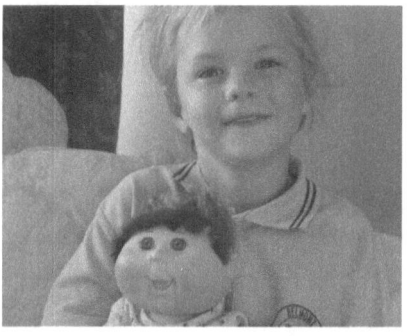

Victoria at home with her doll Sophie

I turned away as I felt the tears start to come. Wow, because Victoria is coping so well, it is easy to forget that she still has to face many things each day, such as the fact that all the girls around her, including me, her sisters and friends have long hair. While her hair is growing, for which we are very grateful to God, on Monday morning before school, she informed me that it wasn't growing fast enough.

Please pray that Victoria will have patience as she waits for her hair to grow and continues to live with the left side weakness.

Friday morning was the first session of hippotherapy. What a wonderful way to finish the week, seeing her so enjoying herself, surrounded by such loving, caring people, all working together to help these children. Victoria herself was thrilled to be there again, and couldn't wait to give Wedge a pat. Please continue to pray that she will be able to attend each hippotherapy session and that there will be improvements in her walking.

On Sunday we had an awesome time at Stockton Beach. The day is organised by Camp Quality, with everything provided by local four wheel driving clubs - cars, lunch, sand boarding. We all had a fantastic day. A special thanks to our driver who made arrangements so we could all travel in one car together, rather than being split into two cars.

It was a very memorable day. Marshall started off the day with a tree climb, while we waited for the car to be set up. Our driver had tea and coffee on hand when we stopped for a break at the Sigma wreck. The next stop was one of the lagoons back in the sand-dunes, part of the Worimi Conservation Lands. A member of the Worimi mob gave a talk about various things made from the bush, bush food and playing the didgeridoo. Marshall volunteered to try some bush tucker. When asked what it tasted like, he tactfully said, 'Mum's cooking.' After lunch it was time for some sand-boarding.

We had a great family day, out enjoying this magnificent country we are so blessed to live in. We are so blessed to be part of an organisation like Camp Quality, who know exactly what families in our situation need to help make it through each day.

Please pray that Victoria will continue to be well despite the chemotherapy treatment, and that her immunity will remain high. And most importantly that she will know the truth of this scripture, no matter where she is or who she is with,

> *Have I not commanded you? Be strong, vigorous, and very courageous. Be not afraid, neither be dismayed, for the Lord your God is with you wherever you go.* (Joshua 1:9)

BLOG POST ON 16TH MAY 2013

Victoria is loving the hippotherapy and enjoying riding on Wedge.

She has been well enough to have chemotherapy both last week and this week. Even though her neutrophils are a bit low, she was allowed to attend a school excursion today to Oakvale Farm and had a great day.

Please pray that Victoria continues to be well, despite the flu season commencing.

A couple of weeks ago when we were having a session with the psychologist in the Paediatric Oncology Department, I noticed this poem by Dorothy Law Nolte on the wall. You may have read this poem before, but I had not seen it before, and thought it was worth sharing.

CHILDREN LEARN WHAT THEY LIVE [33]

*If a child lives with criticism,
he learns to condemn.
If a child lives with hostility,
he learns to fight.
If a child lives with fear,
he learns to be apprehensive.
If a child lives with pity,
he learns to feel sorry for himself.
If a child lives with ridicule,
he learns to be shy.
If a child lives with jealousy,
he learns what envy is.
If a child lives with shame,
he learns to feel guilty.
If a child lives with encouragement,
he learns to be confident.
If a child lives with tolerance,
he learns to be patient.
If a child lives with praise,
he learns to be appreciative.
If a child lives with acceptance,
he learns to love.
If a child lives with approval,
he learns to like himself,
If a child lives with recognition,
he learns that it is good to have a goal.
If a child lives with sharing,
he learns about generosity.*

If a child lives with honesty and fairness,
he learns what truth and justice are.
If a child lives with security,
he learns to have faith in himself and in those about him.
If a child lives with friendliness,
he learns that the world is a nice place in which to live.
If you live with serenity,
your child will live with peace of mind
With what is your child living?

That poem is very thought-provoking, and certainly prompted me to think about some of the less than desirable behaviours I sometimes demonstrate to our children.

And while I know I am very much less than perfect, I thank God for His grace that is readily available to us as parents, and know that this scripture is true for our lives ...

And the grace (unmerited favour and blessing) of our Lord (actually) flowed out superabundantly and beyond measure for me, accompanied by faith and love that are (to be realised) in Christ Jesus.
(1 Timothy 12:14)

Thank you again for your continued prayers, support and encouragement. It is hard to believe that Victoria has now completed forty-five weeks of treatment! We thank God that He has our precious daughter in the palm of His hand.

BLOG POST ON 21ST MAY 2013

Yesterday we got a sniff of another victory regarding Victoria's health and well-being. Praise the Lord. In December last year at an appointment with Vision Australia, I asked if Victoria's loss of left field vision was permanent. The response took a while to come and was very considered, 'You will have to ask the ophthalmic surgeon that question.'

Well, yesterday we had an appointment with the ophthalmic surgeon. He conducted various tests on Victoria's eyes, and then said, 'Her sight has potentially improved.'

I didn't have to ask THAT question. I nearly fell off my chair, and I asked him, 'Do you mean she can now see more things on the left?'

He replied that, 'Some re-learning is possible in children. Their brain can restore this function.'

He was talking about neuroplasticity and other areas of the brain taking over the functions normally performed by the damaged areas. I give praise to our wonderful creator for the way He has created this amazing body we inhabit. Please pray that Victoria's left field vision will continue to improve until it is fully restored.

The doctor also observed, as have the hippotherapy people, that Victoria is compensating for the remaining loss by moving her eyes more, naturally scanning more to the left.

We choose to believe that we will see many more physical victories for Victoria, and we choose to continue to claim 2 Timothy 4:18 over her life.

> [And indeed] the Lord will certainly deliver and draw me to Himself from every assault of evil. He will preserve and bring me safe unto His heavenly kingdom. To Him be the glory forever and ever. Amen. (2 Timothy 4:18)

REFLECTION – THANKFULNESS IS KEY

Reading back through the blog posts in this chapter, I can see that two and a half years later we still have to make the choice continually to look for things to be thankful for.

It would be so easy to only look at the negative things happening in our lives, as they are so obvious. In just these two months of blog posts, we have experienced many less than ideal scenarios.

- Victoria has...

    - had an infection in her leg

    - needed to continue wearing a boot on her left leg each night

    - endured the fasting regime from 7am to around 3pm for the general anaesthetic prior to her MRI

    - had to work through her thoughts about her appearance and how it compares to her friends

    - been almost neutropenic - no immune system

    - missed out on some special events at school

- Victoria and I spent hours and hours waiting in the hospital for appointments and procedures

- we all suffered scan anxiety the weeks leading up to receiving the MRI results

However, we know that to maintain our mental health through all these events we need to find things to be thankful for and keep hope alive. This reminds us that God is with us.

If we search hard enough we can always find something to be thankful for, just like in those initial days when Victoria was diagnosed. So when I reflect on these two months of blog posts, we can also see many things that we have expressed thanks for:

- Victoria

    - The tumour has shrunk by 20%

    - The range of Victoria's ankles has returned to normal, so there is no need to get a splint for her right leg

    - Not losing all her hair, it's starting to grow back

    - Being well enough to have chemotherapy treatment

    - Able to attend a school excursion despite her neutrophil levels

    - Eyesight has potentially improved.

- Camp Quality and the fun experiences they have given our family

- Continued support of extended family

- Living in this magnificent country

- God continually teaching us His ways, for example:

  - Growing in our understanding of our need for more of Him and less of ourselves

  - Learning that He has it all under control; we are not to worry.

  - Understanding that His grace is readily available to us because of Jesus

  - He has Victoria in the palm of His hand.

Looking for things to be thankful for comes easily to me, primarily due to my mother's teachings when I was growing up. While there wasn't a big God focus in our home, my mother always encouraged us to have an attitude of gratitude. After every birthday and Christmas, my sister and I could be found writing thank you letters or making cards. Any act of kindness towards us was always responded to with thanks, either by phone or letter (email wasn't around then). It is an attitude that I have endeavoured to pass on to our children, and they do use emails.

As I said before, being thankful builds hope when all looks hopeless. Each little thing we are grateful for helps us to see that God is in the midst. He hasn't left us alone. When we know that He is there and we can come to a place of trusting as it is written in Romans 8:28, that He is using all these goings on for good. We can take a step of maturity and ask God, 'What are you trying to teach me in this circumstance?'

So, in my daily quiet time with God I started asking Him that question. His answer, 'I am teaching you more about my ways and my love for you, so you will learn to always seek me first.'

In the Gospel of Matthew, Jesus says,

> *Steep your life in God-reality, God-initiative, God-provisions. Don't worry about missing out. You'll find all your everyday human concerns will be met.* (Matthew 6:33 The Message)

But had I not lifted my eyes away from the circumstance and looked for something to be thankful for, I would have missed that opportunity to learn and embrace what God was trying to teach me.

So I encourage you, whatever is happening in your life today, to look purposefully for things to be thankful for, keep your eyes on Jesus, and watch your heart fill with hope. Then take that step of asking God, what are you trying to teach me through this?

Chapter 16

High Temperatures and Hospital Again

BLOG POSTS – 29TH MAY 2013 TO 5TH JUL 2013

BLOG POST ON 29TH MAY 2013

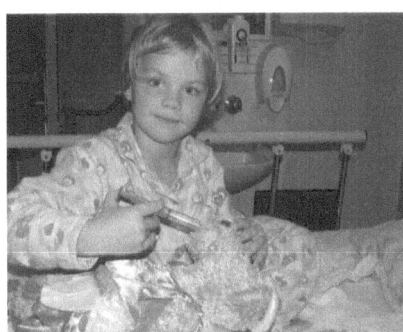

Victoria in John Hunter Children's Hospital giving teddy some medicine

Thank you to everyone who has been praying for Victoria over the past few days. While she is still in hospital, her temperature is now in the normal range. She is washed out and tired.

However there have been some bright spots during the day, such as Victoria having fun doing this procedure on teddy. Victoria also tested out all the bed controls just to make sure they worked correctly.

A big thank you, too, to our marvellous family and friends who have rallied around to help with the other children, especially Ken's parents who sat with Victoria for five hours today so I could have a break and pick up the other children from school.

So once again, despite our circumstances we can find plenty to be thankful for, as The Bible commands us,

> *Give thanks in all circumstances; for this is God's will for you in Christ Jesus.* (1 Thessalonians 5:18 NIV)

Here is another testimony of God's grace. Victoria first became unwell on Monday morning and by the afternoon her temperature was over 38 degrees, which is the trigger for a hospital visit. My wonderful neighbours answered my calls for help, looking after Marshall, Charlotte and Alexandra while I took Victoria to hospital.

I was supposed to be sharing some of our story regarding Victoria at a Biggest Morning Tea for the Cancer Council, at church on Tuesday morning. So I busily made phone calls to find someone to sit with Victoria in hospital so I could go to the morning tea. Another one of my beautiful neighbours graciously made herself available.

HIGH TEMPERATURES AND HOSPITAL AGAIN

However, overnight Victoria's temperature returned to normal, so she was discharged on Tuesday morning. This was fantastic as the early discharge meant both Victoria and I could attend the morning tea. It was such an unexpected blessing having Victoria with me, her presence added a whole other dimension to the talk. She was so well, radiating joy and hope. She 'worked the room' like a professional.

We got home just after midday for a rest. By 3pm, her temperature had risen again, so back to the hospital she went.

As I reflected on the day's activities from the hospital room last night, I was amazed that once again, a situation the enemy had tried to use to create anxiety and disappointment had resulted in such an unexpected blessing. Romans 8:28 is so true,

> *And we know that in all things God works for the good of those who love him, who have been called according to his purpose.* (Romans 8:28 NIV)

Thank you for your support, and please continue to pray that Victoria's temperature will stay down and that she will be infection free.

BLOG POST ON 31ST MAY 2013

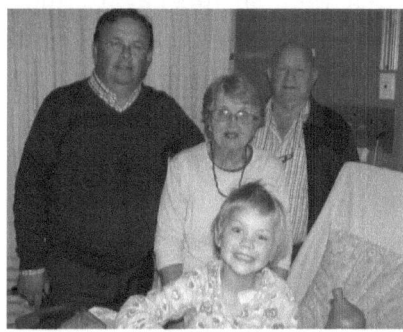

Ken, Nanna, Poppy and Victoria at John Hunter Children's Hospital, J1 ward.

Victoria is home. Thank you to all who prayed for her and practically supported us during this past week.

After a thirteen hour sleep on Wednesday night, she woke up on Thursday morning with more energy and very well rested, rested enough to start on a bit of school work. During the morning, she kept asking what her class would be doing, so with the help of her teacher we 'face-timed' the class. It was great, a real highlight of the day and certainly made Victoria feel connected to what was happening at school.

We had a previously booked appointment with the occupational therapist, so being the wonderfully flexible people they are, they came down to the ward for the therapy session. The bed-sheets will not quite be the same, as the paint came out and went everywhere.

While the therapy session was on, I had the opportunity

to go to a morning tea for parents facilitated by Camp Quality and the paediatric oncology social worker. It was a good opportunity to meet some more parents and share stories, although it was a bit confronting and emotional at times.

Ken and his parents came up to visit again in the afternoon. We received the good news that Victoria could come home, as long as she 'laid low' for a while. The doctor's verdict was that it was a virus, probably just the common cold, that was the cause of this week's drama.

Thank you again to everyone who helped us out or offered to help. Your assistance enabled our week to go as smoothly as possible. And it is another reminder of God's amazing provision for our family in this season.

> *Whom have I in heaven but you? And I have no delight or desire on earth besides you. My flesh and my heart may fail, but God is the Rock and firm strength of my heart and my Portion forever.* (Psalm 73:25-26)

BLOG POST ON 9TH JUNE 2013

It was all go, go, go, this week as Victoria returned to full health. On Monday she had a half day of gymnastics at school. I spent the first half hour of the session crying as I watched Victoria do her best in running relay races. Her teacher so lovingly adjusting the activities Victoria had to do, so she could keep up with the rest of the class.

I think my crying was due to a mixture of the grief and pain that our daughter was different and needed these allowances to be made for her, the appreciation of the loving care so delicately shown for Victoria by her teacher and the continual amazement of the strength of character shown by this little girl who has experienced so much in her five years of life.

In fact, while I was thinking the last thought, I said to myself, if Victoria can participate in these activities, giving it her all with a smile, then surely I can stop crying. So with that thought and a hot chocolate drink given to me by a beautiful sympathetic mum, the tears stopped.

Hippotherapy this week provided another moment for reflection. After Victoria's session, a teenage girl normally arrives in a wheelchair to ride. I didn't know anything about her circumstance until last week when Victoria was in hospital and I saw a newspaper article about her on the noticeboard. She was a pedestrian involved in an accident with a car about two and a half years ago.

This week at RDA she came through the door using a walking frame. Tears again came to my eyes as I could only begin to imagine what it had taken for this girl, and her family, friends and health workers, to achieve this. The resilience and determination of these young people is indeed amazing.

On a slightly different note, but continuing with the teary theme, Friday this week was our fifteenth Wedding Anniversary. We had the opportunity to celebrate by going out for dinner and to a movie. Just to finish off the week with more tears, we chose the movie Song for Marion. I cried through the entire movie, but there was one scene, with one word in particular, that has stuck with me. The word was enjoy.

These things I have seen and thought about this week have made me more determined to just enjoy each moment. What a precious gift it is to be able to enjoy.

> 'Why, you do not even know what will happen tomorrow. What is your life? You are a mist that appears for a little while and then vanishes. Instead, you ought to say, If it is the Lord's will, we will live and do this or that.'
> (James 4:14-15 NIV)

BLOG POST ON 14TH JUNE 2013

It is a year since we found out that Victoria would have to have chemotherapy treatment to stop and hopefully reduce the tumour in her brain. Praise God, the treatment is doing exactly that.

After forty-nine weeks of treatment and with more treatment to come, she is still so full of life. For this we give God the glory.

VICTORIA GRACE

After Victoria had finished chemotherapy treatment this week we explored the fairy garden in the children's hospital. She and Alexandra were fully engaged in exploring the garden and finding all the hidden garden statues.

Victoria has not experienced complete hair loss. Nor has there been the need for a platelet transfusion. Actually, there has been no transfusion of any kind. Please continue to pray that she will remain well for this final four months of treatment.

Please pray for me, this past year of weekly trips to the hospital for either treatment or other appointments has taken a toll emotionally on me. Some weeks all is good, however, yesterday as I reflected on the number of times we have driven to the hospital, sat in the Paediatric Oncology Day Unit, received various news from doctors and stayed overnight in the J1 ward, it all just got too much. It was a struggle to do even the simple things when we got home.

I thought to myself, how am I going to keep this up for another four months? Yes, I know the treatment is working, and Victoria is so well, and I am so grateful for that. But it is the mechanics of doing each day that is getting a bit hard at the moment. And those are the thoughts I went to sleep with.

This morning, when I got up, the first thing I wrote in my journal was 'Dear God, please give me strategies to get through these next four months.' By the end of my devotions time, this was the strategy I had received from God,

> *Steep yourself in God-reality, God-initiative, God provisions. You'll find your everyday human concerns will be met.* (Luke 12:29-32 The Message)

Thank you for your prayers and support, we so need them as we continue to gather strength, wisdom and peace from our God to get through each day, especially me.

BLOG POST ON 23RD JUNE 2013

Last week it was time to say good-bye to Wedge after seven weeks of successful therapy and lots of fun. A big thank you to all the volunteers and Riding for the Disabled staff who made this opportunity possible for Victoria.

As we continue to believe for a great result from her scan on 16 July I have been reflecting on the past two and a half years. This reflection was triggered by a few things that happened this week.

Firstly we continue to experience emotional fallout within our family, which has made for a challenging week. Since Victoria's last hospitalization four weeks ago, one of our children who has seemingly cruised through this whole journey so far, has been really struggling at school. A new challenge begins. Please pray that God gives us wisdom with this situation.

Secondly, I have again had a difficult week emotionally, particularly on Thursday up at the hospital. When I was talking to another mum there, she suggested I needed to get away for at least twenty-four hours. So thanks to help of family and friends that is just what I am going to do on Monday. Please pray that all is well here at home while I am away.

Thirdly I had the opportunity to write a guest blog for ABC Open. The producer asked me to write about how I use the Victoria Grace Conqueror blog and what my aims and objectives were. As I was writing the article I began to think about the benefits I have received from writing about our journey and was quite surprised with what came out of my head and heart. I thank God for this opportunity to share our story and give people another reason to have hope.

All of the events of this week have caused me to think how amazing it is that our family has come this far, and is still hanging together, albeit loosely sometimes. I know I have said it before, but I will say it again, God has definitely been our rock during this journey, and He will continue to be. I think this sentence from Nathan Stone's book, Names of God, sums up well what we have learnt as individuals and as a family.

HIGH TEMPERATURES AND HOSPITAL AGAIN

Man's extremity is ever God's opportunity, not only for deliverance but to teach also wonderful lessons of His purpose as well as providence. [34]

Thank you again for your continuing prayer and support for our family. We are expecting an unexpectedly great result from the MRI on 16th July.

BLOG POST ON 25TH JUNE 2013

The last 48 hours have been very interesting! We have experienced the truth of the scripture,

> *The thief comes only in order to steal and kill and destroy. I came that they may have and enjoy life, and have it in abundance (to the full, till it overflows).* (John 10:10)

The thief had some stealing in mind when on Sunday afternoon Victoria's temperature rose to above 38 degrees, that delightful trigger point for a hospital visit. Ken took Victoria up to the hospital while I readied children and things at home for the impending hospital stay. I was trying to hold back the flood of tears that wanted to come, as this unplanned event was likely to impact on my much needed twenty-four hour break scheduled to commence on Monday morning.

I had completely forgotten how God had so perfectly made a way for me to have this twenty-four hour break.

I was getting into double-mindedness, will it happen? Won't it happen? Rather than trusting that God would make a way through this and there would be abundance.

Sunday night I stayed with Victoria at the hospital. Her neutrophils were good 2.8. Last Thursday they were only 0.7. Victoria's temperature came down and settled all night.

Thank you so much to everyone who prayed for Victoria on Sunday night and Monday morning. When the doctor came around at 10 am she advised that all was well, and Victoria could go home. The plans of the thief had been thwarted once again. Due to Victoria's wellness, I had actually had a wonderful night's sleep in the hospital and a free breakfast. My little twenty-four hour break was turning into a forty-eight hour break. Praise God.

We checked out of Hotel John Hunter as quickly as possible and drove home to get things organised. After taking Victoria to a friend's place I made a bee-line for Merewether Beach for part two of my break. The horrendous weather that had been predicted for days had still not arrived. While there were some dark clouds, the sun still had the victory.

After lunch, I took the opportunity to do a couple of things I used to do in Sydney when I was single, before marriage and children. I used to walk around the beautiful Eastern Suburbs beaches and the Sydney CBD clicking my camera.

HIGH TEMPERATURES AND HOSPITAL AGAIN

It was great to have the time and space to re-live that experience, in a different place that I am really beginning to love.

This past twenty-four hours has been a very restorative time for me, walking, photographing, reading and listening to worship music. Absolute bliss. This morning I awoke at 5.15am and was tempted to turn on the TV to see what the latest news was regarding the inspirational Nelson Mandela. However, at the prompting of the Holy Spirit, instead I started to read the next chapter of the Catherine Marshall book, Something More [35]. She was talking about total relinquishment to God in every area of your life. I then had a break from reading, opened the curtains next to the bed to see the black harbour dotted with lights on wharves and tugs working throughout the night. I turned on my worship music, listened to couple of songs, and then it struck me.

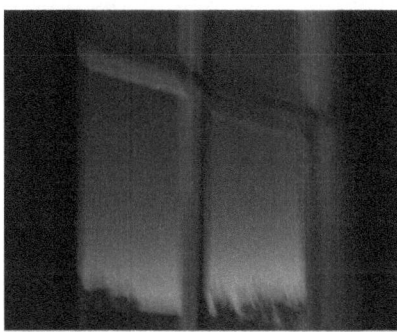

An image of 'The Cross' formed by the window frame in the early hours of the morning at a hotel in Newcastle

I was lying at the foot of The Cross, worshiping Jesus, exactly where He wants me to be, total relinquishment.

Thank you to everyone who has made this break possible. It has been a very blessed time for me. I have life in abundance.

BLOG POST ON 5TH JULY 2013

School holidays are upon us. Last Sunday afternoon, Victoria's temperature started rising, and immediately we started to pray and claim healing in Jesus' name, within an hour she was back to normal. Praise God!

We are now up at One Mile Beach, having a restful holiday in the Camp Quality cabin. Victoria's temperature started rising again yesterday. Again we prayed, claiming healing in Jesus' name, and again within an hour she was back to normal. Praise God! There is no way that we want be going to hospital during this holiday.

We are learning more and more to live out this scripture,

> *No unbelief or distrust made him waver (doubtingly question) concerning the promise of God, but he grew strong and was empowered by faith as he gave praise and glory to God. Fully satisfied and assured that God was able and mighty to keep His word and do what He had promised.* (Romans 4:20-21)

We know that God has promised that,

HIGH TEMPERATURES AND HOSPITAL AGAIN

We are assured and know that [God being a partner in their labour] all things work together and are [fitting into a plan] for good to and for those who love God and are called according to [His] design and purpose. (Romans 8:28)

So we choose to keep in faith for a good result for Victoria's upcoming scan on 16th July. Thank you for standing with us in prayer.

As I have mentioned before, during this treatment period Victoria has not had to have a platelet transfusion, for which we are grateful to God. However the need for transfusions did get me thinking about giving blood and if my veins were suitable, giving plasma and platelets. I used to give blood regularly, first at Uni and then while working. However, since 2006 I somehow haven't found, or made the time to give blood.

I can clearly remember coaxing my sister into giving blood while we were both at The University of Auckland. With our limited knowledge of all things blood, we found ourselves in a state of confusion when we were told we had different blood types, and asking ourselves, was one of us adopted? It was a very nervous wait to get home that night and tentatively ask Mum the question. We were lovingly reassured that neither of us was adopted.

During my twenty-four hours away last week, I drove past

the Red Cross Blood Bank in Newcastle and I thought that is what I will do later on this afternoon, give blood. And so I did, along with a lot of the Newcastle Knights players.

While I was waiting I read about Club Red,

> *Club Red provides an opportunity for organisations and groups across Australia to get together and do something special by regularly donating blood.* [36]

So I have set up a group in Club Red called 'The Conquerors'. If you give blood regularly, or are thinking of giving blood and saving lives please consider joining The Conquerors group. Then every time you donate blood, plasma or platelets, your donation will be attributed to the The Conqueror's group. Our goal is to potentially save 50 lives by 31st December 2013. Just one blood donation can potentially save 3 lives. Let's get giving.

REFLECTION – PRACTICAL TIPS FOR THE HOME OF A CHILD ON CHEMO

Everyone's experience of chemotherapy treatment is different. There are so many variables, including the type of chemotherapy drug, the protocol (amount and frequency that the drug is given) and how the body reacts to the drug. My prayer is that what I share about our experience will assist others when caring for their child, or any other person, who is receiving chemotherapy. These practical tips are based on our experience, so please check with your oncologist before implementing them into your regime.

When you have a child in your home on chemotherapy treatment, it is important to do everything possible to reduce the risk of infection to the child. The child has limited or no immune system to fight infections. For us this meant changing the way we did some things around the home in relation to cleaning, personal hygiene, visitors, medications and equipment we needed to support Victoria's treatment.

Cleaning and personal hygiene

House cleaning is one of my least favourite activities, so this aspect of the journey was a little challenging for me. We had to be hyper-vigilant with both our cleaning and personal hygiene. With the housework, we cleaned the toilets every day using Eucalyptus oil and micro-cloths.

In the kitchen, we had fresh dish-cloths, hand towels and tea towels each day.

Regarding our personal hygiene, hand cleanliness was a big focus. Following the hospital's example, we had Aquim gel pump packs in the kitchen, in the car, in the school bags and in my handbag. In conjunction with this we were very vigilant with hand washing after going to the toilet, before and after eating, and after every nose blow. We had tissue boxes in every room, accompanied by rubbish bins with lids and bin liners, which were emptied every couple of days.

In the bathroom, Victoria had her own hand-towel for wiping her mouth after the mouthwashes. She had a fresh towel every day. And yes, I did have to buy some more hand towels. Also there was no sharing of bath water and bath towels.

Communication with visitors

Some of our visitors were familiar with the importance of reducing the infection risk in our home. But for those who weren't, I made some signs to put at our front door and in the kitchen. This may seem a bit extreme, but when a child who has no immune system gets an infection, their life is at risk. So, in my opinion, it was critical that people who visited our home understood this risk. I also made a sign listing the symptoms to watch for regarding Victoria's health, and the steps to take if any of these symptoms should appear. I love signs, just as much as I love lists.

> *Appendix I – Signs for displaying at home - has examples of the signs I made to display around home, including information signs about infection prevention.*

Another situation arose which I felt warranted a sign. Most of the dog owners that live nearby are very conscientious, picking up their dog's poop and disposing of it appropriately. However, for a period of time, while Victoria was receiving chemotherapy, there was a dog pooping just outside our front gate every day, and the poop was not being picked up. This really infuriated me, so I made a sign asking the offender to pick up the poop and take it with them. I put the sign on our fence. It was very interesting to watch people cross the street in curiosity, read the sign, and observe their faces as they came to the line, 'our child who receives weekly chemotherapy treatment.' The sign worked. We didn't have any more poop at our front gate. An example of this sign is also in Appendix I, just in case anyone reading this book experiences the same problem.

Medications

The chemotherapy treatment meant there was the need for additional medicines to be taken at home. Here is an example of what Victoria had to take.

- Bactrim – An antibiotic, a pre-emptive measure to fight off infections

- Nilstat – A mouthwash, to help prevent mouth ulcers

- Bi-carbonate Soda – A mouthwash, to help prevent mouth ulcers

- Ondansetron – An anti-nausea drug

Victoria's medicine box also included:

- Lactrolos – to help reduce constipation, although eventually we found the most effective way to reduce constipation was putting the timer on continually for 30 minutes, and getting her to drink at least half a cup of water when the timer went off.

- Kenalog – a great paste for covering mouth ulcers.

HIGH TEMPERATURES AND HOSPITAL AGAIN

> *Initially for my own reminder, but then also for anyone who was looking after the children while Ken and I were out, I made some signs relating to Victoria's mouth-care and medications. These were in the bathroom and kitchen.*
>
> *Examples of these signs are in Appendix I – Signs for displaying at home.*

Equipment

We had to make sure we were properly equipped to accurately determine if Victoria was febrile and needed to go to hospital, so we invested in an infra-red ear thermometer, along with a box of alcohol wipes. Using this thermometer was a lot quicker than the under-arm digital thermometer, and was more accurate. We soon got into the habit of taking the temperature three times in the same ear, just to check that the temperature was rising. We didn't want to make an unnecessary trip to hospital.

I set up a box called 'Victoria's medicines etc.' It contained the thermometer, alcohol wipes, anti-nausea medicine, mouthwashes, mouth ulcer cream, Lactrolos and other medications (e.g. Bactrim). It also had a black sparkly bag with the local anaesthetic cream, tape, scissors, plastic covering and the digital under-arm thermometer. These items were needed for making sure Victoria's port was ready to be accessed, either before receiving chemotherapy, or when she became febrile. We would take the black sparkly bag with us wherever we went; just in-case she became unwell while we were out and about.

> *Appendix J has a list of the contents of the Medical box I put together for Victoria.*

Another piece of equipment we had around the house was God's Word, just as it says to do in Deuteronomy.

> *Therefore you shall lay up these words of mine in your heart and in your soul, and bind them as a sign on your hand, and they shall be as frontlets between your eyes. You shall teach them to your children, speaking of them when you sit in your house, when you walk by the way, when you lie down, and when you rise up. And you shall write them on the doorposts of your house and on your gates, that your days and the days of your children may be multiplied in the land of which the LORD swore to your fathers to give them, like the days of the heavens about the earth.* (Deuteronomy 11:18-21 NKJV)

HIGH TEMPERATURES AND HOSPITAL AGAIN

We had scriptures on the walls and cupboards in the kitchen, in our bedrooms and in the toilets, all declaring God's goodness and faithfulness. We wielded His Word as a weapon in this fight for our child's life. Here are some of the scriptures from our upstairs toilet door.

> *Now faith is confidence in what we hope for and assurance about what we do not see.* (Hebrews 11:1 NIV)

> *Our help is in the name of the LORD, who made Heaven and earth.* (Psalm 124:8 NKJV)

> *Let us draw near to God … Let us hold unswervingly to the hope we profess, for He who promised is faithful.* (Hebrews 10:22-23 NIV)

This is not a comprehensive list of all the things that need to be done around the home if you have a child on chemotherapy. It is just some of the things that we found useful to have around our home for the fifteen months when Victoria was receiving treatment. As I said at the beginning of this section, I know that everyone's experiences with chemotherapy are different. My prayer is that these tips will be of some help and be a catalyst for other actions that can help reduce the risk of infection in your home.

Chapter 17

Precious Family Time

BLOG POSTS – 12TH JUL TO 26TH JUL 2013

BLOG POST ON 12TH JULY 2013

We give thanks to God and all the people who donate to Camp Quality, as we have just enjoyed a very relaxing holiday at One Mile Beach. It is just sooooooooooooo good to get away from the house and be at the beach.

Victoria took on the challenge of riding a new bike. Her catch-cry throughout the holiday was, 'If Marshall can do it, and Charlotte can do it, and Alexandra can do it, then I can do it.'

Victoria's physio advised that with the left-side weakness it will be more difficult for her to learn to ride a bike without training wheels. So could you please pray that she will have the perseverance to achieve this childhood milestone.

Thank you to everyone who has helped us out over the last month. You have all made a huge difference to our lives. The practical help has certainly eased the pressure I have been feeling and has returned my emotional state to a more even keel. For those of you who read this blog and don't live near-by, I am going to mention some of the practical help that we have received in this past month, to illustrate how loving and caring people in this world can be, and to encourage you to help a family near you who is in need.

- ✓ Mum and Dad, funded my twenty-four hour break at a beautiful hotel

- ✓ My sister and family, funded the room service I received during my twenty-four hour break

- ✓ Friends who looked after the children so I could have the twenty-four hour break

- ✓ Friends and teachers from school who arranged for our house to be cleaned twice during the school holidays

- ✓ Thursday 'chemo' day meal roster - friends and teachers from school bring dinner to our home on Thursday, when I am often emotionally spent

- ✓ A friend who does my shopping for me when it is just too difficult to get to the shops - sometimes getting just milk and bread is a huge help

PRECIOUS FAMILY TIME

- ✓ Friends who have looked after Marshall, Charlotte and Alexandra during the chemotherapy treatment in the holidays as the hospital advised that they didn't want siblings in the treatment room these holidays

- ✓ Friends who have stepped in to be pseudo Aunts and Uncles and great role models for our children

- ✓ Family, neighbours and friends who are 'on call' to help out at home at a moment's notice if Victoria is required to go to hospital

We are so grateful to every one of you, and to those who have helped us that I have not mentioned. Thank you for being so generous with your love, time and finance.

Thank you, too, to everyone who has joined The Conqueror's blood donating group. If you want to join please go to the Red Cross Australia website. The goal is 50 potential lives saved by 31st December 2013.

Finally and most importantly thank you to everyone who is praying for us. We are so grateful that Victoria is so well and that our holiday was not interrupted with an emergency hospital visit. Victoria had chemo yesterday, week fifty-three.

Please continue to pray that the scan results next week will be extremely positive, just like this beautiful courageous girl.

And please pray that we can continue to stand strong in our faith, as in Romans,

> *No unbelief or distrust made him waver (doubtingly question) concerning the promise of God, but he grew strong and was empowered by faith as he gave praise and glory to God. Fully satisfied and assured that God was able and mighty to do what He had promised. (Romans 4:20-21)*

BLOG POST ON 13TH JULY 2013

As the day begins and I prepare myself mentally to live in victory in every moment of this day, another day of fasting for Victoria, a general anaesthetic and her eleventh MRI scheduled for 2pm, it is Psalm 103 that God has led me to this morning.

> *Bless (affectionately, gratefully praise) the Lord, O my soul; and all that is [deepest] within me, bless His holy name!*
>
> *Bless (affectionately, gratefully praise) the Lord, O my soul, and forget not [one of] all His benefits -*
>
> *Who forgives [every one of] all your iniquities, Who heals [each one of] all your diseases,*
>
> *Who redeems your life from the pit and corruption,*

PRECIOUS FAMILY TIME

Who beautifies, dignifies, and crowns you with loving-kindness and tender mercy;

Who satisfies your mouth [your necessity and desire at your personal age and situation] with good so that your youth, renewed, is like the eagle's [strong, overcoming, soaring]!

The Lord executes righteousness and justice [not for me only, but] for all who are oppressed.

He made known His ways [of righteousness and justice] to Moses, His acts to the children of Israel.

The Lord is merciful and gracious, slow to anger and plenteous in mercy and loving-kindness.

He will not always chide or be contending, neither will He keep His anger forever or hold a grudge.

He has not dealt with us after our sins nor rewarded us according to our iniquities.

For as the heavens are high above the earth, so great are His mercy and loving-kindness toward those who reverently and worshipfully fear Him.

As far as the east is from the west, so far has He removed our transgressions from us.

As a father who loves and pities his children, so the Lord loves and pities those who fear Him [with reverence, worship and awe].

For He knows our frame, He [earnestly] remembers and imprints [on His heart] that we are dust.

As for man, his days are as grass; as a flower of the field, so he flourishes.

For the wind passes over it and it is gone, and its place shall know it no more.

But the mercy and loving-kindness of the Lord are from everlasting to everlasting upon those who reverently and worshipfully fear Him, and His righteousness is to children's children.

To such as keep His covenant [hearing, receiving, loving, and obeying it] and to those who [earnestly] remember His commandments to do them [imprinting them on their hearts].

The Lord has established his throne in the heavens, and His kingdom rules over all.

Bless (affectionately, gratefully, praise) the Lord, all you His hosts, you His ministers who do His pleasure.

PRECIOUS FAMILY TIME

Bless the Lord, all His works in all places of His dominion; bless (affectionately, gratefully praise) the Lord O my soul!
(Psalm 103)

BLOG POST ON 18TH JULY 2013

Thank you to everyone who has prayed for Victoria. God is faithful. The tumour has not grown. It is stable, possibly slightly reduced in size.

It has taken me a good twenty-four hours to come to a place of heartfelt thankfulness for this result. I had hoped for a reduction like we witnessed in the April scan. However, that is not the case this time. This morning I found solace in Psalm 23:6.

Surely or only goodness, mercy and unfailing love shall follow me all the days of my life, and through the length of my days the house of the Lord [and His presence] shall be my dwelling place.
(Psalm 23:6)

The chemotherapy treatment will continue another three months until October. Please pray that Victoria will continue to handle this treatment so well with minimal side effects, and that all hospital visits will be a positive experience for her.

Thank you to everyone who prayed for Victoria on the

day of the MRI. She had to fast from 7am. The MRI which was originally scheduled for 2pm did not take place until 5.15pm. Victoria coped very well with this delay, with minimal complaints regarding hunger or thirst. We thank God for the peace that was over her. The nursing staff commented on how good she had been with the delay.

We spent our time alternating between painting in the Starlight Express room, and watching DVDs on my laptop. It was a long day. A big thank you to everyone who has helped out this week, looking after our other children while Victoria and I went to the various appointments.

In the midst of all the scan and doctor's appointments this week, the news came through that the Starlight Children's Foundation have granted Victoria's wish. Victoria's wish is to go to the snow and throw snowballs at everyone. So on Sunday 4th August, our whole family is off to Mt Buller in Victoria, for five nights. Everything is paid for by the Starlight Children's Foundation; travel, accommodation, meals, ski gear hire, lift passes and ski lessons. This is such an amazing opportunity for Victoria and our family. It will certainly help these next three months pass more quickly. We are so grateful to all the Starlight Children's Foundations' sponsors and people who have donated to this fantastic charity.

Thank you again for the prayers and support that are offered to our family. It all truly helps us to make it through each day.

PRECIOUS FAMILY TIME

BLOG POST ON 20TH JULY 2013

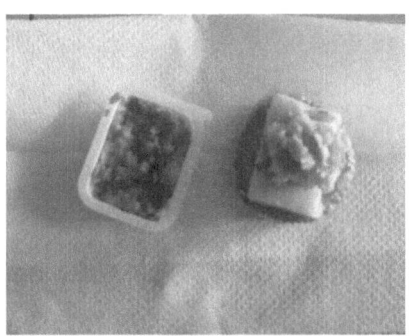

Victoria's creations with hospital food at John Hunter Children's Hospital, J1 ward.

Presenting food creations from the John Hunter Hospital. Here is Victoria's latest creation. All you need is two crackers, cheese, plum jam and margarine.

Yes, that's right, Victoria had a high temperature late yesterday afternoon, so up to John Hunter Hospital we went. She is doing a lot better today, and will hopefully go home tomorrow.

Please pray that:

- ♥ Victoria's neutrophils and haemoglobin increase as they were quite low last night

- ♥ Victoria is well enough to start term three of school on Monday

In my recent daily devotions, God has been reminding me to put on His armour. Ephesians 6:13-18, particularly verse 16,

> *Lift up over all the [covering] shield of saving faith, upon which you can quench all the flaming missiles of the wicked [one].* (Ephesians 6:16)

Thank you for continuing to lift up Victoria and our family. Thank you, too, to everyone who has helped our family this weekend.

BLOG POST ON 21ST JULY 2013

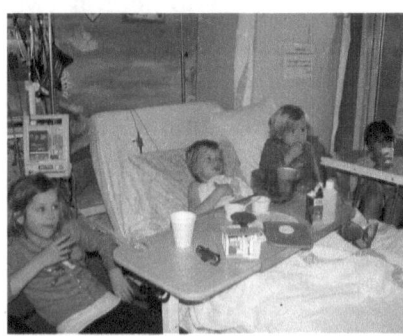

Charlotte, Victoria, Alexandra and Marshall at John Hunter Children's Hospital, J1 ward

Victoria is looking a lot better this morning. Her blood results are healthier and she has been given the all clear to go home. Thank you for your prayers and for the support we have received throughout the weekend.

Yesterday aside from making food creations, Victoria had a visit from Jasper, from Delta Therapy Dogs. It was a highlight of the afternoon. He is such a beautiful dog.

PRECIOUS FAMILY TIME

Ken brought up the other children for a visit too. Victoria was pleased to see them. They were pleased to see the Nickelodeon channel on the TV as we don't offer that service at home.

These two days of forced rest have done both Victoria and me a lot of good. Victoria is looking rested for school tomorrow. I have had time to get my head around all I heard last week from the doctors and to seek God to see what He has to say about it. Here are some of the scriptures He gave me this morning, to stand on over the next three months. I hope they are encouraging to you, too, for whatever trials you are currently facing in your life:

Casting the whole of your care [all your anxieties, all your worries, all your concerns, once and for all] on Him, for He cares for you affectionately and cares about you watchfully. (1 Peter 5:7)

The Lord will give [unyielding and impenetrable] strength to His people; the Lord will bless His people with peace. (Psalm 29:11)

Blessed be the Lord, who bears our burdens and carries us day by day, even the God of our salvation! Selah [pause and calmly think of that]! (Psalm 68:19)

VICTORIA GRACE

For with God nothing is ever impossible and no word from God shall be without power or impossible fulfilment. (Luke 1:37)

BLOG POST ON 25TH JULY 2013

Thank you to everyone who has been praying for Victoria over the past few days. As some of you already know she has been back in hospital since Tuesday night this week, with high temperatures, cause is unknown. Her temperature is stable today, but she is still not back to the joyful Victoria we know and love.

A very big thank you to my sister who has extended her visit from New Zealand to look after the other children at home, thus giving Ken's parents and our friends some respite.

Every Thursday fortnight Camp Quality and the hospital social worker for families of kids with cancer, put on a yummy morning tea for the parents with kids currently in the J1 ward. The morning tea was on this morning. It was a blessing to leave the hospital room and chat with some of the other parents. It is always confronting to listen to what the other parents are experiencing with their children, however at the same time supportive as we all have some understanding as to what each other is going through.

PRECIOUS FAMILY TIME

On Tuesday morning as I was doing my devotions I read this scripture,

> *When Jesus looked out and saw that a large crowd had arrived, he said to Philip, 'Where can we buy bread to feed these people?' He said this to stretch Philip's faith. He already knew what He was going to do.* (John 6:4-5 The Message)

As I read this scripture, the last part of the passage, 'He already knew what He was going to do' really spoke to my heart. I felt that God was telling me that He already knows the outcome with Victoria's health, and I am to rest in that truth. The situation is not out-of-control. How necessary it was for me to have that assurance in my heart prior to coming to hospital late Tuesday night. Once again I am so grateful to have a God who is the creator of the universe, and yet so interested in our individual well-being.

Please pray that Victoria's health will continue to improve.

BLOG POST ON 26TH JULY 2013

Victoria has been given the ok to check out of Hotel John Hunter today. Praise God! We are now looking forward to ten days of perfect health before we hit the snow at Mt.Buller.

The turning point for Victoria yesterday was the arrival at the hospital of her sister Alexandra and Aunty Allison and Jade, who have been doing a sterling job back at the house.

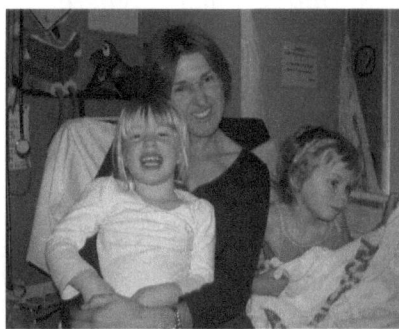

Jade, Allison and Victoria at John Hunter Children's Hospital, J1 ward

Until their visit, Victoria had no interest in eating, drinking or taking her medicine. And there were certainly no smiles. The love of family can do amazing things. The smile hasn't left Victoria's face since their visit. A friend visited later in the afternoon and they busied themselves making airline tickets for the snow trip while I had a little break.

Later in the evening the wonderful Starlight Children's Foundation volunteer that has been assigned to our family visited Victoria. She has played a key role in the planning of Victoria's wish and helping us get prepared. A friend of hers gave Victoria a blow-up penguin just to help us get into the 'snow mood' a bit more.

Please pray that Victoria will remain well for the next three weeks while we prepare for the wish, and experience the wish. After a bit of reading last night I found out that the week we are at Mt.Buller is Christmas week, so there are numerous extra activities going on there. What a blessing!

Once again these past three days have been a strong reminder that wrapping myself in God's word is key to mentally getting through the difficult times.

> *And He humbled you and allowed you to hunger and fed you with manna which you did not know nor did your father know that He might make you recognize and personally know that man does not live by bread only, but man lives by every word that proceeds out of the mouth of the Lord.* (Deuteronomy 8:3)

Thank you again to everyone who has been praying for Victoria and our family. We appreciate your faithfulness more than I can say.

REFLECTION – THE BIBLE

During this journey, my love for The Bible has grown tremendously. In the seven blog posts of this chapter, there are ten passages of Scripture that God put on my heart to share. Four of them came from the Psalms. Reading these scriptures gives me hope for the future. They remind me that God is always with us, and He has given us all we need.

The Bible is not a book of stories from the long ago. It is literally God-breathed. It is our Heavenly Father's instruction book for us to live by.

> *Every Scripture is God-breathed (given by His inspiration) and profitable for instruction, for reproof and conviction of sin, for correction of error and discipline in obedience, [and] for training in righteousness (in holy living, in conformity to God's will in thought, purpose and action), so that the man of God may be complete and proficient, well fitted and thoroughly equipped for every good work.*
> (2 Timothy 3:16-17)

God's word has been a constant for me throughout this journey, always there in the day and in the night. The wisdom in it has helped guide me through each day, helping me to direct my focus back to Jesus regardless of what is happening around me. Psalm 119:105 says it this way,

PRECIOUS FAMILY TIME

Your word is a lamp to my feet and a light to my path.
(Psalm 119:105)

Prior to Victoria's diagnosis, I read the bible and journaled most days. Although often I was reading from a place of 'a good Christian reads their Bible every day.' It was something on my daily jobs list. I definitely learned something every time I read God's word, but it was a very different experience to what happens now when I read God's word.

Over the years God's word has become more and more central to my well-being and a guide in my life. I believe you can see this change as you read through the emails and blog posts. There has been a shift from looking at circumstances the world's way, to starting to see them more from God's perspective, well, in the small way that a human can.

This shift started from a place of desperation. In a practical sense it began with me searching for solace in God's word, devouring the Psalms with their alternating emotions of fear and hopelessness, then faith and trust. I could completely relate to the passages where the Psalmist felt abandoned, and then in the next few lines described the victory God had given him. The Psalms were like my new best friend. It was as though through them God was saying to me, 'I understand how you are feeling.' And of course, He was saying that. He does know completely how we feel. He experienced suffering in the death of His Son Jesus.

Now when I wake up in the morning, there is a desire in me to sit quietly and read His word, before I do anything else in our busy household of six. I know I need to give my Heavenly Father an opportunity to speak to me about the day, before I embark on my daily activities. Being receptive to what God is showing me through what I am reading, is one way I can learn how He wants me to go about my day. It is a time of surrendering my plans and listening to His plans.

Now whenever I open my Bible, I have an expectation God will speak to me through His word. And no matter how long I spend reading and talking with God, I always get some direction, sometimes for the whole day, sometimes for the next few minutes, but it is enough to know I am in His will.

Reading the bible first thing in the morning, also gives me the encouragement I need emotionally, as per my reference regarding the Psalms. His words of life build hope in me, and help me to understand that I am loved, I truly am a child of God, and that God has a good plan for my life and my family's life. Over time He has also drawn me to scriptures for other people that I have connection with. What a privilege to be a vessel of God's encouragement and love.

God's word gives us promises that we can declare with our mouths. As I have mentioned before, the words we speak are critical to our well-being regardless of our circumstance. Furthermore when they are declared in the authority of Jesus' Name they have the power to change our circumstance. As Joel Osteen reminds us,

> *Proverbs 18:21 says, 'Life and death are in the power of our tongue.' What are you saying about your future? What are you saying about your family? What are you saying about your finances? Make sure the words you are sending out are in the direction you want your life to go.* [37]

One of my prayers when writing this book has been that God would use it to show people how His word can give you the strength, day by day, to get through a difficult time. So I encourage you to find some quiet time each day, sit and ask God to speak to you through His word. Open your bible, be expectant and wait to hear that still, small voice. He loves you. He has things He wants you to do. He will speak to you.

> *Every part of Scripture is God-breathed and useful one way or another – showing us truth, exposing our rebellion, correcting our mistakes, training us to live God's way. Through the Word we are put together and shaped up for the tasks God has for us.*
> (2 Timothy 3:16-17 The Message)

Chapter 18

The Wish

BLOG POSTS – 3RD AUG TO 9TH AUG 2013

BLOG POST ON 3RD AUGUST 2013

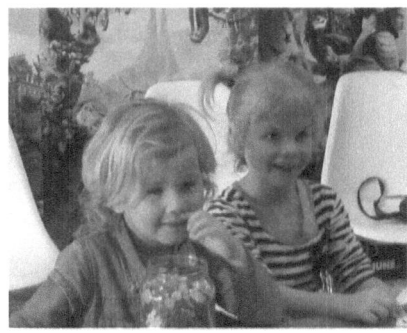

Alexandra and Victoria in the Starlight Express Room at John Hunter Children's Hospital when Victoria's Starlight Wish was granted.

This is the look on Victoria's face at the Starlight Express Room this week when she was given a surprise presentation of her Wish. It was a priceless moment. Her wish-granter was there with a basket of necessary snow things.

As we witnessed this celebration I reflected on everything Victoria has been through and overcome and how wonderful it is that she is now getting this 'wish'. It is hers and hers alone. While the rest of our family is getting to experience Victoria's wish too, we have gently reminded the children why Victoria has received this wish, and that we need to do our very best to celebrate her and where she is at today.

We are so grateful to God that we are all well, and this week has been such a contrast to last week. Thank you to everyone who has been praying for the health of Victoria and our family. Please continue to pray for good health and that Victoria's wish will be the best experience ever for her.

This Psalm came to mind this morning.

> *It is good to give thanks to the Lord, and to sing praises to Your name, O Most High; To declare Your lovingkindness in the morning, and Your faithfulness every night.* (Psalm 92:1-2 NKJV)

Victoria has been enjoying the Transition to Riding program at the Riding for the Disabled Centre, doing different exercises to improve her balance, and learning how to give instructions to Sprinkles. This week she started riding in a saddle, with stirrups and reigns. It is all very exciting, and continues to be a highlight of each week.

Throughout the huge highs and lows of this journey, there

is one thing that I have endeavoured to keep consistent in my life, and that is a daily handing over of Victoria to God. Some days that has been harder than others. Some days there has simply been no other choice. I have found this passage of scripture to be the absolute truth.

> *Come to Me, all you who labour and are heavy laden and overburdened, and I will cause you to rest. [I will ease and relieve and refresh your souls.] Take my yoke upon you and learn of Me, for I am gentle (meek) and humble (lowly) in heart, and you will find rest (relief, ease and refreshment and recreation and blessed quiet) for your souls. For my yoke is wholesome (useful, good - not harsh, hard, sharp or pressing, but comfortable, gracious and pleasant) and My burden is light and easy to be borne.* (Matthew 11:28-30)

BLOG POST ON 4TH AUGUST 2013

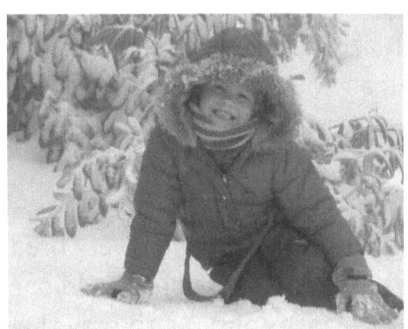

Victoria sitting in the snow at Mount Buller, Victoria

This photo says it all. We made it. After a shaky start on Saturday, with Alexandra at the doctors early in the morning, we finally left for Sydney at about 4pm. The Starlight Children's Foundation kindly added a travel day to either end of our trip, including a night's accommodation in Sydney. They have been so thoughtful and thorough with everything to ensure Victoria has the best experience possible. This extra night certainly made the travel a lot easier.

Today, Sunday, was a big travel day, leaving Sydney on a 7am flight for Melbourne. We took all possible precautions with Victoria. There was no way she was not going to get to the snow. Upon arriving in Melbourne we got the Mt Buller Ski Express for the three hour drive to Mt.Buller. We were certainly not disappointed as we drove up the mountain and the children got their first glimpse of the snow. There were plenty of squeals of delight in the coach. There was 15cm of snow today.

The Starlight Children's Foundation arranged accommodation at an amazing hotel. After checking out the hotel, it took us about an hour to get kitted up for the snow, and then out we went exploring. Marshall thought it would be fun to eat the snow.

It has been such an awesome day. Everyone is very tired, but full of great memories already. Thank you to everyone who has 'prayed us here'. Please continue to pray that everyone remains well and Alexandra's cold will not spread to anyone else.

We are so absolutely grateful to the Starlight Children's Foundation for granting Victoria her wish. It was just so precious to see her jumping, sliding and rolling in the snow today.

It is movie month in September for the Starlight Children's Foundation. They are featuring Victoria's story to encourage people to get involved in fundraising during movie month. If you want to know more about it, please go to their website.

BLOG POST ON 6TH AUGUST 2013

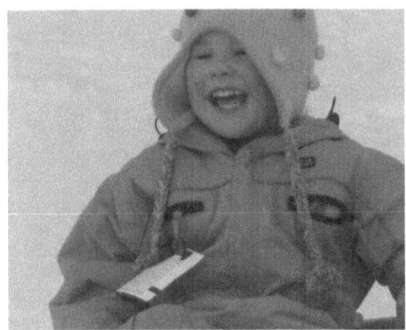

Alexandra on the toboggan at Mount Buller, Victoria

And the photo of the day goes to Alexandra. We have had two great days in the snow, on the snow and exploring the beautiful Mt.Buller. Thank you to everyone who has been continuing to pray for us, as you can see by this photo Alexandra is now feeling on top of the world.

We again give thanks to God for this amazing opportunity for our family. We are certainly creating many great family memories, memories that will be talked about for many years to come.

> *I will praise You, O Lord, with my whole heart; I will show forth (recount and tell aloud) all Your marvellous works and wonderful deeds! I will rejoice in You and be in high spirits; I will sing praise to Your name, O Most High.* (Psalm 9:1-2 NKJV)

BLOG POST ON 9TH AUGUST 2013

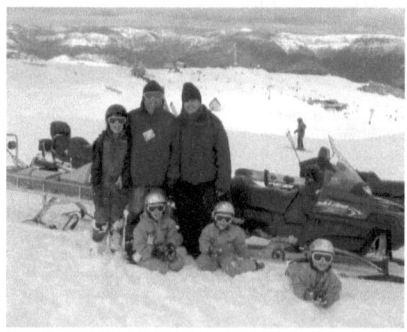

Robinson family at the summit of Mt Buller, Victoria

We have had two more amazing days at Mt.Buller. Yesterday we were treated to a Ski-doo ride to the summit, courtesy of Mt Buller Guest Services. Here we are with the amazing view of the Victorian Alps behind us. How spoilt we are.

It is hard to believe that our week here is almost over.

THE WISH

Victoria has enjoyed every moment of her wish. I think one of her favourite activities has been lying down and rolling in the snow.

I heard Victoria say to Ken earlier in the week,

'Daddy, I would really like to live in the snow.'

We have been surprised at how much she absolutely loves the snow. Victoria definitely knew her own heart when she asked to go to the snow for her wish. We will be leaving Mt Buller with so many wonderful family memories, and knowing that despite our circumstances, God is always in the midst. We have experienced His favour.

> *Blessed and enviably happy [with a happiness produced by the experience of God's favour and especially conditioned by the revelation of His matchless grace] are those who mourn, for they shall be comforted.* (Matthew 5:4)

While, by the grace of God, Victoria is still with us here on earth, we have mourned for what she has lost and been through. And while we would never have asked for these circumstances, we have experienced a part of God's character that we probably wouldn't have otherwise. Joyce Meyer's commentary about this verse explains further.

In Matthew 5:4, Jesus said that those who mourn are blessed and that they will be comforted. The comfort of God which is administered by His Holy Spirit, is so awesome that it is almost worth having a problem just to be able to experience it. As with most of the things of God, it goes far beyond any kind of ordinary comfort. Let God be your source of comfort. When you are hurting, just ask Him to comfort you. Then wait in His presence while He works in your heart and emotions. He will not fail you. [38]

Thank you again to everyone who has continued to pray for us. Everyone is still 100% healthy, Praise God.

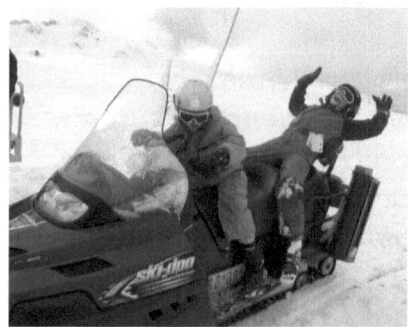

The real Ski-doo drivers at the summit of Mt Buller, Victoria

REFLECTION – CHARITIES

Through the hospital social worker, we found out about many wonderful charities that exist to help families with seriously ill children. These organisations have unique missions, tailored to meet the diverse needs of a family at different times along their journey.

The financial assistance we received from these organisations helped us significantly. In the preceding years, we'd used up all our reserves to keep our business afloat during the global financial crisis. It was a relief to know that all our utility bills, and even some of our mortgage payments, would be covered by these charities.

As I have written in my blog, the camps, retreats and family fun days provided fabulous opportunities for each of us to have some time out from the constant stress of the cancer journey; how we met new people, build our resilience by trying new things, and sometimes just rested. They helped revive us emotionally. I have realised that stable mental health, is a key component in sustaining our family life during this long season.

The wish that Victoria received from the Starlight Children's Foundation, was a totally different realm of giving. The preparation that was put into the wish granting process by our wish-granter was very thorough. At every step there were checks to ensure that the wish was what Victoria wanted, and that she was not being influenced by anyone else in the family. The four month lead up to the wish gave Victoria so much to look forward to, helping to take the focus off the chemotherapy treatment.

Many family memories were created during that week at the snow, some so hilarious that they are still spoken about with laughter today. It was an experience that we as a family could not have given Victoria, due to our financial constraints. We are so grateful to the Starlight Children's Foundation Australia who generously provided an amazing family experience in the midst of suffering.

I mentioned most of the charities that have helped us in my blog posts, with the goal of communicating the great work they do.

> *Appendix K gives a brief summary of the assistance we received from various charities.*

It is very humbling to be on the receiving end of such marvellous help. The generosity of businesses and people who give their money and time, enabling these programs and facilities to become a reality, is quite overwhelming.

Every time we went to a supermarket that was raising

money for Redkite, I would just cry when I saw the wall near the check-out counters filled with all the little cards that people had purchased for $2.

When I was feeling brave enough, I would say to the check-out person, 'We are one of the families who benefit from all those donations.'

On one of those occassions, one of the check-out people replied saying, 'Really, it is so good to actually meet someone who receives from a charity.'

Sometimes a conversation about our journey would follow, depending on how many people were in the checkout queue. I would always buy at least four of the donation cards, one for each of our children.

Many of these charities do not receive any government funding, so if you feel led to donate to one or more of them (or an equivalent organisation in your country), I know your donation would be greatly appreciated and will tangibly help a child and their family. In Australia, these charities are all registered with the Australian Charities and Not-for-profits Commission (ACNC), the independent regulator of charities.

While donations to registered charities are tax deductible, there are many other benefits you can receive from donating to charities. Mary McCoy on moneycrashers.com cites ten other benefits. Here are two of them.

Activating the Reward Centre in your brain. *A study by a University of Oregon professor and his colleagues demonstrates that charitable contributions create a response in the brain that mimics one activated by drugs and other stimuli. This response elicits a surge of dopamine and endorphins that are experienced as "hedonic" and rewarding. Charitable giving can feel pleasurable in the deepest parts of your physiology – more so than a night on the town or a new outfit.*

Improve life satisfaction. *A German study provides ample evidence that people who give more to others – in both time and resources – experience greater satisfaction in life than people who do not. In fact, communities of people with high levels of giving tend to demonstrate greater satisfaction within the community than groups of people who do not give generously. Essentially, you're going to be happier in your community if it's made up of folks who give to one another.* [39]

Originally though, giving to others was God's idea. In The Bible, He tells us to share what we have with others.

> *But if anyone has this world's goods (resources for sustaining life) and sees his brother and fellow believer in need, yet closes his heart of compassion against him, how can the love of God live and remain in him? Little children, let*

> us not love [merely] in theory or in speech but
> in deed and in truth (in practice and in sincerity).
> (1 John 3:17-18)

And, God gives us the best example of giving, when He gave His Son, Jesus, to die for us, so that our relationship with Him could be restored and we could have eternal life in heaven.

> For God so loved the world that He gave His
> only begotten Son, that whoever believes in
> Him should not perish but have everlasting life.
> (John 3:16 NKJV)

We all have something we can give - money, time, skills or things, like toys. For example, Marshall donated his almost new toys to the Ronald MacDonald House Charities. We just need to take time to open our eyes and see, and open our ears and listen. We can all do something practical to meet the needs of others, whether it is your neighbour, seriously ill children and their families, refugees, indigenous communities, or communities in the developing and third world. We are not here on earth forever. We can't take our money and our possessions with us when we die and go to heaven. So let's all use what we have been blessed with, to help others.

Chapter 19

Reality Hits Fast

BLOG POSTS – 11TH AUG TO 19TH SEP 2013

BLOG POST ON 11TH AUGUST 2013

It didn't take long for reality to set in once we returned home from our wonderful trip for Victoria's wish. We arrived back home at 3pm on Saturday, and by 8pm that night she started to feel unwell. By 6am Sunday morning we were on our way to the John Hunter Hospital. After some initial blood tests showed that she had plenty of neutrophils, and the absence of any more high temperatures, it was decided at 10am that Victoria could go home.

However at 10.30am when the nurse came to de-access her port, it was apparent that her temperature was climbing again, so home was no longer an option. Hence we are still here and will be at least until tomorrow.

Victoria is okay within herself, and certainly brightened up with a visit from the rest of the family this afternoon. We are just all so grateful that she remained well while on her wish, another example of God's amazing grace on her life.

Today has certainly been a day for drawing deep from God's strength.

> *Behold, God is my salvation! I will trust and not be afraid, for YAH, the LORD is my strength and song; He also has become my salvation. Therefore with joy will you draw water from the wells of salvation.* (Isaiah 12:2-3 NKJV)

I know I say this on every update, and I am going to keep saying it, thank you so much for your prayers and practical support. Please don't underestimate the power of your prayer. Our whole family is a testimony to answered prayer, and every single bit of practical help given to us helps us to all keep going physically and emotionally. Thank you, thank you, thank you.

BLOG POST ON 12TH AUGUST 2013

The doctor advised this morning that Victoria will need to stay in hospital for most of today, and will be reviewed again this afternoon. She is well within herself, and has managed to do some spelling this morning. The hospital school teacher brought down some air-drying clay for her to model with. Thanks for continuing to uphold her in your prayers.

REALITY HITS FAST

For anyone who is interested, here is the general process that happens when Victoria has to come into hospital with a high temperature.

We have pre-packed hospital bags at home for Victoria and I, sort of like the bag you prepare for hospital for the impending birth of a baby. Victoria's bag includes a few pairs of pyjamas'; some of her favourite books, including Angels watching over me [40], given to her by her Prep teachers last year; some of her favourite toys, like little plastic figurines that she plays imaginary games with; and a change of clothes to wear when she is discharged.

My bag is mainly filled with electronic gadgets to enable to me to keep communicating with the outside world. Chargers for my mobile phone, laptop, wireless modem, photo chip reader etc. I have a folder in which I keep all my current paperwork for our business, so I can just grab that when we need to go, as sometimes there are ideal conditions in hospital for getting a lot of bookwork done. I have also realised after the last couple of visits, that there is potentially the opportunity to do a few self-beauty treatments such as pre-packed facials and hair conditioning, so will be on the look-out for some of those this week to put in my bag.

We also have another bag, the foodie bag. The hospital provides Victoria with food however I have to provide my own. So I bring some Uncle Toby's porridge sachets, bananas and my Tupperware heating container and that takes care of breakfast. Around lunch-time I am normally ready to have a break from the hospital room, so take a walk down to the cafeteria for a wrap of some sort. For dinner I have been enjoying some of the more exotic Healthy Choice frozen meals, followed by a chocolate bar from the fundraising box at the nurses' station.

Now back to the process... When Victoria's temperature reaches the trigger point of 38, we phone the J1 ward at the John Hunter Hospital and advise them of what is happening.

At home we then put the anaesthetic cream on Victoria's port. It takes about 30 minutes for the anaesthetic cream to work. It takes us about 30 minutes to get to the hospital, so it means that Victoria's port can be accessed as soon as we arrive at hospital, and the blood can be taken to find out her blood count and some put aside to see if a bacterial infection is present.

When we get to the hospital, we go directly to the J1 oncology ward, by-passing the Emergency Department. Normally we go into the treatment room in J1 where the nurse does the accessing, and a doctor comes to do an initial assessment. Once those tasks are done, Victoria can go to her assigned room. These are all single rooms with their own bathroom, TV, PlayStation and a parent bed for me or Ken to sleep in.

Sometimes, depending on varying factors, the doctors

will decide to start antibiotics via the port, or they wait to see what transpires. And then we pray and wait.

Now that Victoria is at school, when she is well enough, she normally gets a visit around 9am from the school teacher who plans out some activities for the day.

And that is generally how it all happens. As for what happens back at home while Victoria is in hospital, that is another story for another day.

BLOG POST ON 13TH AUGUST 2013

Last night, at about 9pm, Victoria announced that she had some itchy spots on her leg. I had a look at it and thought, not good. We buzzed the nurse, who buzzed the doctor. The verdict was chicken pox. So it was off to the special isolation room.

Neither Victoria nor I can leave this room. I had to ask the nurse to make my porridge for me this morning, which she happily did. The nurses wear masks when they come in to see Victoria.

When I was talking to my mum this morning, I said I no longer have any expectations about how each day will go. However on reflection this is not entirely true, I do have one expectation, and that is that God will get us through each day. He has in the past and I believe He will today, and He will in the future.

VICTORIA GRACE

The Bible verse I read this morning for my devotions provides hope for the day and the future

> But unto you who revere and worshipfully fear My name shall the Sun of Righteousness arise with healing in His wings and His beams and you shall go forth and gambol like calves [released] from the stall and leap for you. (Malachi 4:2)

We have just seen the oncologist who has confirmed that Victoria has chicken pox. At this stage she only has four spots on her leg, so hopefully no more will appear. She will be going home this morning, no chemo this week, no school this week and no horse-riding this week, just at home keeping a very low profile.

A friend text me Psalm 91 while we were waiting to see the doctor this morning. I am holding on to these promises.

> 'If you'll hold on to me for dear life', says GOD, 'I'll get you out of any trouble. I'll give you the best of care if you'll only get to know and trust me. Call me and I'll answer, be at your side in bad times; I'll rescue you, then throw you a party. I'll give you a long life, give you a long drink of salvation!' (Psalm 91:14-16 The Message)

Thanks for your continuing prayers and support.

BLOG POST ON 23RD AUGUST 2013

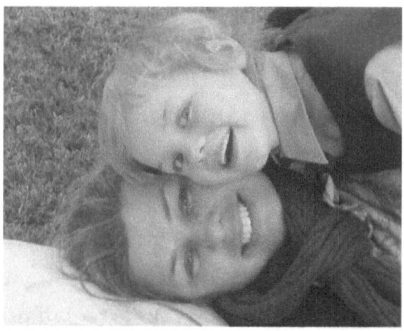

Wendy and Victoria on the grass at home

Do you think we are mother and daughter?

Thank you for all your prayers. Victoria is doing very well. The chicken pox did not progress beyond the four spots, and it did not progress beyond Victoria, Hallelujah, praise the Lord.

Victoria was excited to be back at school on Tuesday, with her friends and beautiful teacher. On the way home from chemo yesterday she said, 'Mum, I just love school.'

Victoria's blood count was high enough yesterday for her to have chemo, and she has enough platelets to go riding today. Yippee.

If you have been following our journey for a while you will know that we have a huge number of people who support our family in many different ways. One place we receive a lot of support from is the local church that we belong to. In the media the church often gets very bad press, and understandably so for some of the events that have occurred. However, there is another side to the church, a loving, caring, supportive side, that doesn't seem to get very much press at all. In fact I can't remember the last time I read a positive article about the church in the newspaper or watched a news item on television. So here is something positive about being part of a church family.

When it became evident to me in June that I was struggling emotionally with the weekly visits to the hospital, I shared my feelings with a couple of close friends. One of whom is a member of the church we attend. Within a couple of weeks the church had assigned someone to give me and our family the extra practical support we needed to make it through the last few months of this round of chemo.

I was finding it harder and harder to go to the hospital each week with a positive attitude. I was just plain tired of it all. I did not want my negative attitude to rub off on Victoria or Alexandra, as they both looked forward to the hospital visits. Thirteen months on, they still skip down the hospital corridors saying hello to everyone. Praise God. I decided I needed someone with me to share the load. Ken had to work - he was not an option. My immediate family all live in NZ - they were not an option. So our church family stepped in and filled the gap. They set up a roster of people to come up to the hospital with us on Thursdays, which means I can often go and have a quiet lunch by myself, not having to rush back to the treatment room.

Another area in which we desperately needed additional support was our marriage. Marriage can be difficult enough sometimes, without the added pressures of having a seriously ill child. Ken and I have been very much in survival mode for the past two and a half years, and now as Victoria's treatment is coming to an end, we thought it was time to start to reconnect as a couple and re-build our marriage as we move into this next phase of this long journey. But our problem was getting time alone. With four children and running our own business, there is always someone or something that needs attention. Once again our church family has stepped in to fill this gap, organizing a babysitting roster for each Saturday night for the next few months. Ken and I had our first date night last Saturday night. The date only lasted an hour as we were simply exhausted, but it was great to get out and actually be able to finish a conversation without being interrupted.

So I hope you can see that being part of a church family has been such a blessing to our family. They have filled the gaps in our lives many times. The church is not perfect, but it can be a very loving and caring organisation that does its very best to show Christ's love. Our family is a testimony of that love.

> *This is love; not that we loved God, but that he loved us and sent his Son as an atoning sacrifice for our sins. Dear friends, since God so loved us, we also ought to love one another. No one has*

ever seen God; but if we love one another, God lives in us and his love is made complete in us. (1 John 4:10-12 NIV)

For anyone who is interested, the church we belong to is Macquarie Life Church, Cardiff, NSW.

BLOG POST ON 31ST AUGUST 2013

Praise God for a 'normal' week. Victoria was well enough to have chemo on Thursday. She enjoyed a good week at school, culminating with an exciting outdoor ride through the sensory garden at Riding for the Disabled on a glorious Friday afternoon. The sensory garden is full of things that the children can look at and touch as they ride through the garden.

Next week will be Victoria's last riding session for the year. We are so grateful that she has been given this opportunity, and are extremely grateful to the volunteers who give up their time to make these programs possible. Hopefully Victoria will be able to do more riding programs next year.

Regarding chemotherapy, the current program is for chemo to continue until the end of October. Victoria continues to have minimal side effects from the chemotherapy. We have dramatically increased her daily water intake which has stemmed the constipation problem that she was experiencing. Not sure why it took twelve months to work that out. Her next scan is Tuesday October 22nd.

Thank you for your continued prayers and support. It is such an encouragement to us all to know that we are not doing this journey alone. A friend gave me this scripture through the week, a reminder of our Heavenly Father promises.

> *Whatever God has promised gets stamped with the Yes of Jesus. In him, this is what we preach and pray, the great Amen. God's Yes and our Yes together gloriously evident. God affirms us, making us a sure thing in Christ, putting his Yes within us. By his Spirit he has stamped us with his eternal pledge - a sure beginning of what he is destined to complete.* (2 Corinthians 1:20 -22 The Message)

BLOG POST ON 10TH SEPTEMBER 2013

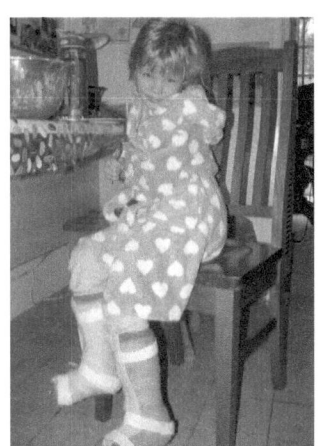

Victoria at home with the night boots on

Victoria has remained well since having chemo last week, week three in the four week program. Over the past three months, it has been after the week three treatment that Victoria has ended up in hospital with high temperatures, so we are very grateful that this has not been the case this past week.

Before the chemotherapy last week, Victoria had some new night boots made. She chose green and gold.

We had great fun on Father's Day and Ken's birthday which were one and the same day this year. All home and well, well enough to get out on our boat, Mistral 2, for the afternoon. A very different picture to the same time last year when Victoria was in hospital. Again we are ever so much more grateful for these precious moments together as a family.

Yesterday was Marshall's birthday, and he wanted to have takeaway pizza for dinner. When the pizzas arrived, guess whose photo and story was on the box topper - Victoria's - advertising the Starlight Children's Foundation movie month, a fundraising event. Please go to their website if you want to find out how you can participate and help raise money for this wonderful charity, from which our family has greatly benefited.

It is amazing the difference it has made to us all not having had Victoria in hospital for over three weeks. For me, I feel that I am not in "catch up" mode around the house and with the other children, as has pretty much been the case for the past three months. We are praying that between now and the end of October when the treatment finishes, that Victoria will indeed continue to be well.

We give God the praise and glory for His continual hand on our family, in every area of our lives.

> *Blessed be the Lord, because He has heard the voice of my supplications. The Lord is my Strength and my [impenetrable] Shield; my heart trusts in, relies on, and confidently leans on Him, and I am helped; therefore my heart greatly rejoices, and with my song will I praise Him. The Lord is their [unyielding] Strength, and He is the Stronghold of salvation to [me] His anointed. Save Your people and bless Your heritage, nourish and shepherd them and carry them forever.* (Psalm 28:6-9)

Please continue to pray that Victoria will remain well, and the next scan on 22nd October will give a good report. Many, many thanks.

BLOG POST ON 19TH SEPTEMBER 2013

Victoria was well enough to have chemo today, week sixty-two done and dusted. We also had an appointment with the OT who was pleased with the way Victoria was using pressure from her left hand to stabilise the paper when writing. When chemo finishes we may look at some more hydrotherapy to help build strength in her left arm.

A big thank you to everyone who is 'carrying' us through Victoria's last 3 months of treatment. It is so re-assuring and comforting to know that we have this support. Ken and I have been enjoying our Saturday night date nights, getting out and having that uninterrupted conversation. The Thursday hospital help has made a huge difference to my mental state, even as I drive into the carpark, I think to myself, 'I have help. This will be a good day.'

The Thursday night dinners that arrive at our home, finish off a huge day wonderfully. And of course everyone who is praying for our family, thank you, thank you, thank you.

Another big thank you to everyone, family and friends, who made it possible for me to get away for a night earlier this week. This time alone gave me the opportunity to pray and gather my thoughts regarding making an emotionally healthy transition from treatment life to a more normal life for hopefully at least twelve months. The wonderful Redkite organisation run a transition group via telephone, a telegroup, for seven weeks. Redkite describes the group this way,

> *These intimate discussions bring parents together and reduce the sense of isolation they can often feel once they return to the community. They*

> *provide the opportunity for everyone to share their experiences and learn from each other, encouraging the development of personal strengths and coping skills.* [41]

Unfortunately I won't have the opportunity to join one of these groups until early 2014, so I really wanted to take some time to consider the changes that will take place in our lives when Victoria finishes treatment at the end of October and how we can best manage that change. Somethings won't change, for example Victoria will still have the portacath in, so the routine of going to hospital if she has a high temperature will still be required. But as she won't be having chemotherapy pummelling her neutrophils, she should be at less risk of an infection, and hopefully the hospital visits will be as simple as checking her out and sending her home again. Rather than the three day stay.

During this transition time, one area we do want to focus on is re-building the connections within our family. By the grace of God they have withstood the barrage of change and upheaval over the past almost three years. But now it is time to move from survival mode, back to doing, what Ian Grant in his book Growing Great Boys calls 'Intentional parenting'. Here is an excerpt from his book...

> *During the sixties and seventies, a generation of parents who'd rebelled against societal norms and the standards of their parents began*

experimenting with different ways to bring up their kids. A relatively values-free approach to child rearing became the norm for many. However, as children who have grown up without boundaries are picking up the pieces of their sometimes chaotic lives, there appears to be a bit of a swing back. Educators and parents recognise the value of mentoring, boundaries and a sense of future as passed on by loving and firm parents. I like to call this 'intentional parenting'. [42]

While I was away for the night I was finally able to finish reading this book, and it has given me many ideas about re-connecting with our children. I will mention a few over the coming weeks.

To finish off this post, here is a poem from the book. You may have seen it before, but I think it is well worth another read, especially given the way today's society generally works.

>THE ANYWAY POEM [43]
>By Kent M. Keith
>
>*People are often unreasonable, illogical, and self-centred*
>*Forgive them anyway*
>*If you are kind, people may accuse you of selfish, ulterior motives*
>*Be kind anyway.*

REALITY HITS FAST

If you are successful, you may win some false friends and some true enemies
Succeed anyway.
If you are honest and frank, people may cheat you.
Be honest and frank anyway.
Transparency may make you vulnerable.
Be transparent anyway.
If you find serenity and happiness, others may be jealous.
Be happy anyway.
What you spend years building may be destroyed overnight.
Build anyway.
The good you do today may be forgotten tomorrow.
Do good anyway.
People who really want help may attack you if you help them.
Help them anyway.
Give the world the best you have and it may never be enough.
Give the world your best anyway.
You see, in the final analysis, it is between you and God.
It was never between you and them anyway.

REFLECTION – KEEPING THE LEFT LEG WORKING

Before Victoria could be discharged after the brain surgery she had to have a review with a physiotherapist. At the time, I didn't fully understand the necessity of this appointment and had absolutely no idea that physiotherapy would become such an important part of Victoria's life. This was to be the first of many appointments aimed at keeping her left leg as functional as possible, and to learn how to take good care of her left foot. As one therapist said to Victoria, 'You only get one left foot, so you need to take care of it.'

In this reflection, I have sought to explain some of the actions we have taken, and continue to take, to keep Victoria's left leg and foot growing in both size and strength. As with the shoulder, arm and hand, we have learnt that it is not sufficient to do the exercises for six weeks and then stop. From our experience, there needs to be purposeful action every few days It is exactly as the orthopaedic surgeon advised, 'She needs to use it or lose it'.

Physiotherapy and Hydrotherapy

Victoria's first physiotherapy regime involved weekly visits for reviews of her gait. Movement was the main therapy we did at home, keeping her active and using the muscles in both legs. Walking up and down stairs was a particularly beneficial exercise and thankfully our house has stairs.

Six weeks after the brain surgery Victoria was given the all clear to go swimming again. This meant she could start hydrotherapy sessions. These worked on both upper and lower limbs. Victoria's love for the water, combined with an excellent physiotherapist, meant these were always lots of fun. Her strength and range of movement steadily improved.

Ankle-Foot-Orthosis (AFO)

After the hydrotherapy, during a review of Victoria's leg and ankle, the physiotherapist decided that even though there had been some improvement in her balance and leg strength, an AFO (Ankle Foot Orthotic – a leg and ankle brace) was required. The wearing of the AFO would provide Victoria with more stability when walking. That is, it would enable her to move around more safely by reducing the number of falls. The AFO is the splint Victoria wears on her left leg.

Hippotherapy

About fourteen months after surgery Victoria was given the opportunity to join the hippotherapy program at our local Riding for the Disabled centre. Hippotherapy is basically physiotherapy on a horse. Victoria thoroughly enjoyed the ten-week program. It helped strengthen her core muscles, and left limbs. She completed another hippotherapy program the following year, 2013.

Horse Riding

At the end of the second hippotherapy program, Victoria participated in the Transition to Riding program. She then continued on with the riding programs in 2014 and 2015. These programs helped her to continue gaining core strength, all in a beautiful environment out of the hospital setting. They also helped her grow in confidence as she could see the progress she was making each week. Eventually she was able to walk off-lead, without a helper leading the horse, and trot on-lead.

Hydrotherapy

Over the years Victoria has done a few six week blocks of hydrotherapy. These times of intensive therapy have had positive effects on her muscle strength and range. They also helped to increase her physical endurance. Initially the sessions lasted 25 minutes, however by the end of the six weeks they were lasting for an hour. One physiotherapist provided us with some instruction sheets of the exercises used in Victoria's hydrotherapy sessions. We laminated them and in the summer months Victoria uses them as a guide for exercising when she is in our pool.

Regular sustained stretching

Daily stretches - As Victoria has grown, regular sustained stretching has been introduced to her routine every two or three days. These stretches prevent the muscles from tightening and shortening, eventually becoming less effective. They are essentially a twenty minute stretch of the left hamstring muscle, and a twenty minute stretch of the left calf muscle.

Wedge and variable height desk – To assist with the calf muscle stretches we purchased a stretching wedge, a wooden box with a top that slopes at 45 degrees. The lower end of the wedge butts against wall. When Victoria stands on the wedge with the back of her legs and heels against the wall, she achieves a good stretch in her calf muscles. Often her left calf muscle is so tight she is unable to have her heel against the wall without experiencing a huge amount of pain. At those times Victoria moves her foot up the slope of the box until it is in a less painful position.

To help Victoria maintain the stretch we borrowed Ken's small variable height desk. He had purchased the desk a few years earlier for use with his laptop. We were able to adjust the desk height so that Victoria could work at or play on her ipad, while she was stretching. This worked so well, that now during school term both the wedge and the variable desk live at the back of her classroom. This means that if she is having pain in her leg at school, she can take her school work to the variable desk, stand on the wedge and continue to stretch her calf muscle. Thus she continues on with school work with minimal disruption. She takes off her splint when using the wedge.

Night-boots - The daily sustained stretching is complemented by Victoria wearing a boot on her left leg, sometimes on both legs, during the night while she sleeps. The boot is made in a stretch position, so the calf muscle gets at least a ten hour stretch while Victoria is sleeping. Due to the heat, this can be very uncomfortable in the summer months. We have found that sprinkling talcum powder inside the boot is a great way to reduce heat rash.

Serial casting – At one period Victoria had serial casting on her left leg. This is when a cast is made while the leg and ankle are in the stretch position. It is worn for a week or so. Then, depending on the ankle range achieved, another cast may be made for a further week, and the process is repeated until the desired range achieved.

Swimming

Victoria's love of swimming has been a blessing to her physical and emotional well-being. Unlike walking, swimming requires her to use all four limbs to keep moving forward, helping them all to grow in strength, increase range of movement, and build core strength. Her desire to swim competitively makes her work hard to achieve new personal best times. This has again helped to give her more confidence in what her body can do.

> *Over the years we have learned much about hemiplegia, the condition that among other things, impacts on the bones and muscles on the left side of Victoria's body.*
>
> *Appendix B has a basic medical explanation of hemiplegia.*
>
> *Appendix C and D have some of Victoria's upper and lower limb therapy activities.*
>
> *Appendix L has a list of some of the equipment we have purchased to help with therapy.*

Thanking Jesus' for His healing power

While we are doing all the recommended physiological actions to help improve Victoria's left side, we are also continually thanking Jesus for His healing power at work in her body. We know that physical healings happened when Jesus walked on the earth.

> *And Jesus went on from there and passed along the shore of the Sea of Galilee. Then He went up into the hills and kept sitting there. And a great multitude came to Him, bringing with them*

> the lame, the maimed, the blind, the dumb, and many others, and they put them down at His feet; and He cured them, so that the crowd was amazed when they saw the dumb speaking, the maimed made whole, the lame walking, and the blind seeing; and they recognised and praised and thanked and glorified the God of Israel. (Matthew 15:29-31)

And we can expect to see these things and more, now, here on earth as Jesus says,

> I assure you, most solemnly I tell you, if anyone steadfastly believes in Me, he will himself be able to do the things that I do; and he will do even greater things than these, because I go to the Father. (John 14:12)

Derek Prince, with his leg-lengthening ministry has witnessed the physical healing power of Jesus in many people's lives, many times over. His book, God's Word Heals [44], is full of these stories, as well as some great teaching on healing God's way.

My prayer is that this reflection is helpful to those readers who care for people suffering from hemiplegia, as well as an encouragement to have faith that Jesus' healing power is still available today.

Chapter 20

Living From a Place of Victory

BLOG POSTS – 27TH SEP TO 29TH OCT 2013

BLOG POST ON 27TH SEPTEMBER 2013

Victoria was well enough to have chemo yesterday. The count-down is on now. The current plan is four more treatments. This may possibly change to only three depending on the MRI results we get on 28th October.

Victoria herself is very well, just a bit tired, so school holidays have come at a good time for her. This week the Newcastle Star had an article about the fundraising event Starlight Movie Month, which has now been extended to end of October. The article included some of Victoria's story and the amazing support she has received from the Starlight Children's Foundation.

Thank you again to everyone who is helping us get through these last six weeks. It is all making a huge difference to our family.

We continue to choose to trust God for a good report from this next scan. We thank our God for the way that Victoria has coped with this circumstance and overcome all the challenges she has had to face. We thank our God that our family has learnt so many good things over the past few years and has been so humbled by the love and support we have been shown by so many people.

> *He is the Rock, His work is perfect, for all His ways are law and justice. A God of faithfulness without breach or deviation, just and right is He. (Deuteronomy 32:4)*

BLOG POST ON 3RD OCTOBER 2013

This morning when I woke up I felt overcome with emotion at the thought of going up to the hospital again for Victoria's treatment. Here is the scripture from my morning devotion.

> *I am with you all the days (perpetually, uniformly, and on every occasion), to the [very] close and consummation of the age. Amen (so let it be). (Matthew 28:20)*

These were the exact words I needed to hear, and have placed in my heart. I was so distraught I could hardly have a conversation on the phone with my wonderful friend who was bringing us dinner tonight. I thought to myself how am I going to do this for another three weeks?

Eventually I made it to the shower and took some deep breaths, and felt more able to face the day.

Thankfully a friend from church was going to look after the other children today, so it would just be Victoria and I at the hospital today. Once again, I am so grateful for all the support church has provided us with, especially in the last three months.

Finally Victoria and I made it to the hospital. She had her port accessed, and then the doctor nonchalantly said, 'This will be the last treatment today and we will re-assess after the scan.'

I just sat there a bit stunned, that was not the plan last week. All I could think was, Thank you God, you knew this had to be the last day.

We had the support of another wonderful friend from church with us at the hospital today. In fact when she arrived, I left her with Victoria and just went off to have a good cry - tears of relief and joy.

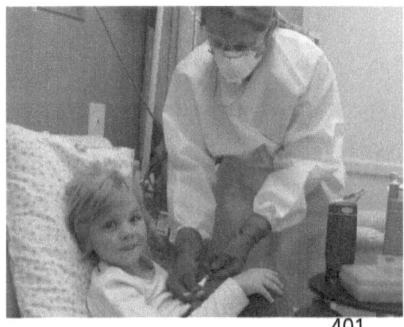

Victoria receiving her last chemotherapy treatment at the Paediatric Oncology Day Unit at John Hunter Children's Hospital

Here is Victoria getting ready to have chemo, with one of the very caring nurses that we are again so grateful for.

A couple of months ago, Victoria had asked if she could have some goldfish when chemo finished. So as soon as chemo was finished today, we picked up Alexandra and Charlotte, and went to the pet shop. Ken and Marshall met us there. What excitement in the shop.

First Victoria picked out the bowl and all the decorations. Next step was to pick out three fish. Victoria named them immediately: Amy, Emily and Grace. It was so exciting.

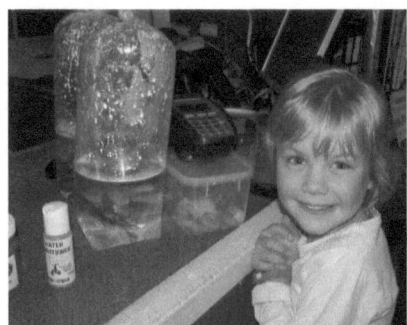

Victoria buying her fish at a local pet shop

After a careful drive home, the fish bowl was set up, the fish put in, and Victoria gave them their first meal.

What a day it has been; a morning of despair and complete reliance on God to get me through each moment; an afternoon of joy knowing that we have a time ahead of us where we can be normal family again. And joy at seeing Victoria loving her fish.

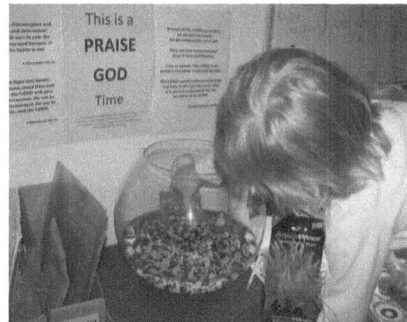

Victoria setting up her fish tank at home

You may have noticed a pink sign at Victoria's desk saying, 'This is a Praise God time.' That sign has been up in our house since Victoria came home from having brain surgery in January 2011. It has been a constant reminder to me that God is in control even when it doesn't feel like He is, and that He has a plan, and it is always right and good. Indeed His plan for today was right and good.

Thank you again to everyone who has helped us in so many different ways. Words really cannot express our gratitude. Please continue to pray for us as we wait for Victoria's scan on 22nd October and results on 28th October.

BLOG POST ON 18TH OCTOBER 2013

Two weeks has passed since Victoria finished chemo. Despite having her temperature climb the day after she finished treatment, thankfully peaking just below the trigger point, Victoria continues to do well. Thank you for continuing to lift her up in prayer.

VICTORIA GRACE

The night after treatment finished we had a celebration dinner at home. Based on what I had read in the Growing Great Boys [45] I had three discussion points for dinner time.

1. Everyone to share a specific example of how well Victoria had met the challenge of fifteen months of weekly treatments.

2. Victoria to share how each person in the family had helped her during treatment

3. Everyone in the family to share something positive that had come from Victoria being unwell.

Needless to say the discussion that came from these questions was very insightful.

Because treatment was stopped earlier than anticipated, Victoria was thrilled to be able to spend the whole day at school with her friends for her birthday.

These past two weeks have been like living in a dream, with no hospital visits for treatment and fewer concerns about illness. Victoria has been able to enjoy two weeks uninterrupted at school.

At home we have been able to do some jobs that really needed doing with the help of my mum and dad visiting from NZ.

For me, it has also been a very emotional time, with tears coming anytime, anywhere. The supermarket seems to be a favourite place for them to turn up. The psychologist tells me it is very normal after holding everything together for such a long time, and that I should just let them come out and make sure I get some rest.

There are a few reasons for the tears. Firstly I get very overwhelmed when I think of the huge number of people who have helped us in so many different ways since January 2011. The kindness and grace people have shown our family is a testimony to God's goodness. Secondly I grieve for Victoria, while she has been amazing throughout this time, her childhood is not as it should have been.

Thirdly, in faith we know Victoria's future is good, however as a mum walking through this daily it is tough. The latest lot of vitamins I am taking are called Mums Rescue - how appropriate. I am struggling with the thought of going to the hospital next week for Victoria's three monthly MRI. Thankfully once again God has provided support with my mum being here and friends to come up and help us through that long day.

Thank you again for your faithfulness and prayers. Our main prayer points currently are:

- ♥ Victoria will remain well to have the general anaesthetic next Tuesday for the MRI

- ♥ I will have the emotional strength to do the MRI day well for Victoria's sake

- ♥ The results of the MRI will be positive

This morning I gained such encouragement from,

> *Know, recognize and understand therefore that the Lord your God, He is God, the faithful God, Who keeps covenant and steadfast love and mercy with those who love Him and keep His commandments to a thousand generations. (Deuteronomy 7:9)*

I know that as it says in Nehemiah 8:10, the joy of the Lord will be my strength today

BLOG POST ON 22ND OCTOBER 2013

Thank you to everyone who has been praying for us this past week, including today. Thank you, too, to everyone who emailed and texted messages of support and encouragement today. They all helped us to get through the day with a smile.

Victoria's MRI was very uneventful. Everything ran like clockwork. Her MRI was scheduled earlier than normal, which meant we were home just after 5pm.

It was such a blessing to have mum and my friend Lorna

with us today for extra support. Their presence really helped me to keep my mind focused on the moment, rather than running away with unhelpful thoughts.

We continue to believe for a good outcome of this MRI. We know that God has Victoria in His hands. He is in charge, as He reminded me this morning when I read my bible,

> *Know, recognize and understand therefore this day and turn your [mind and] heart to it that the Lord is God in the heavens above and upon the earth beneath; there is no other.* (Deuteronomy 4:39)

We get the results of the MRI on Monday 28th October.

BLOG POST ON 29TH OCTOBER 2013

We met with Victoria's oncologist yesterday who advised that the MRI indicated the tumour is stable. It has not gotten bigger, for which we are very grateful. The chemotherapy has done its job well, and God has ensured our beautiful daughter has had minimal suffering throughout the last 15 months of treatment. Again, we are very grateful for His goodness and faithfulness.

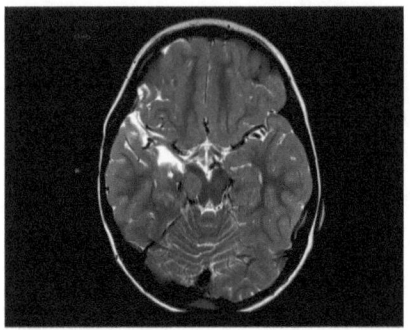

MRI of the tumour in Victoria's brain on 22nd October 2013

The plan going forward is to watch and wait. Victoria will have another MRI in February 2014, when again the situation will be re-assessed. So for three months at least her body will get a break too, and we can all enjoy the encroaching Christmas holidays without having to be in a hyper-vigilant state.

Thank you again to everyone who has prayed and/or practically supported us over these recent years. I often marvel at the 'shape' our family is in now, given all it has been through, and know that your prayers and support have been absolutely essential to our well-being. Thank you for being such faithful family and friends.

Despite the circumstances we have faced, we have continually been blessed throughout this time. This weekend our entire family was blessed when we attended a Camp Quality Family Camp at the Great Aussie Bush Camp at Tea Gardens. We all had the opportunity to get out of our comfort zones.

Victoria and I pushed the boundaries by going on the flying fox. Well at least I did, Victoria was quite calm about it. The launching platform was quite high. But we did it and I certainly screamed the loudest of the group. It proved little challenge for Marshall and likewise for Charlotte, who both managed to get about three goes each.

Next it was on to the mud pit, which I declined to do. But again Marshall, Charlotte and Victoria took up the challenge. The Great Aussie Bush Camp staff were fantastic, helping the children and encouraging them to give everything a try. Marshall was in boy heaven. Charlotte pushed on through, determined to do whatever Marshall was doing. Choice - over or under, Marshall chose under, Charlotte chose over, sensible girl. And Victoria walked around.

Sunday morning proved to be Ken's biggest challenge - a dolphin cruise on the beautiful Port Stephens. I wasn't sure if he could handle the coffee and relaxing. The children took the opportunity to play in the boom net off the side of the boat. Once again the staff helped Victoria so she could join in the fun too. They were marvellous. Alexandra had fun watching from the boat.

Alexandra did challenge herself by doing rock climbing on the Saturday afternoon, and making it up to the 'red line'. Unfortunately I didn't get any photos as Camp Quality treated all us parents to an afternoon at nearby Tea Gardens. It was great to spend time together as a couple and then hang out with other parents that we now have so much in common with. Camp Quality certainly hits the mark 100% when it comes to supporting children and their families. It is organisations like Camp Quality that again have made a huge contribution to helping our family be where we are today. We are so grateful to them and all their supporters.

As I have said many, many times before, Jesus is the Rock I stand on, and will continue to stand on as we enjoy the next three months, and prepare for the journey ahead, whatever it may hold. For now, we embrace today.

> *The Lord is my Rock, my Fortress, and my Deliverer; my God, my keen and firm Strength in Whom I will trust and take refuge, my Shield, and the Horn of my salvation, my High Tower.* (Psalm 18:2)

FINAL REFLECTION – THREE YEARS OF LEARNING

So here we are, almost three years on from when Victoria was diagnosed with a brain tumour. From a physical perspective, she has had brain surgery, hundreds of hours of physical therapies and completed fifteen months of chemotherapy. At the end of those fifteen months, at the review appointment the oncologist advised that within another twelve months chemotherapy treatment would probably recommence.

At least for now we have time to take a breath and reconnect as a family. Emotional healing needs to take place in each of us as we have lived these past three years in survival mode. We have to re-learn how to be a family without having a child on chemotherapy.

In the back of our minds there is that question, what will the next scan show? It is a battle to remain in faith, believing that God is for us and that He has this situation under control. We still choose to believe that God's healing power will manifest in Victoria's body.

God has brought our family through so much, and has taught us so many things in these past tumultuous three years. We have learned a little about the intricacies of the wonderful human body that He designed and created. He has shown us things about ourselves, our family, people and of course Himself.

We have learned that when the difficult seasons come we need people around us. Each individual (family and friends), professional (doctors, nurses, therapists and counsellors), organisation and community (church, school, neighbours and charities) has had a different role to play, but they are all necessary. I have learned that it is important to stay connected, and not to get isolated, as tempting as that may be. The physical, emotional and spiritual implications of isolation are too great.

One of my goals in writing this book is to show the importance of reaching out to people in the difficult seasons, asking for help, and graciously receiving help when it's offered. Our family would not have come through this journey as well as it has without the love and support of family, friends, neighbours, church community, school community and charities. Had it not been for this support we probably would have lost our home and our marriage, and all been deeply emotionally scarred from this experience.

We have been reminded of the importance of running to God in the difficult seasons, rather than running away from Him. Our need for Him becomes even greater in times of crisis, not as a crutch, but rather as a Rock to stand on and re-build our lives.

Here are some of the specific lessons God has taught me on this journey:

God's grace is sufficient

And He said to me, "My grace is sufficient for you, for My strength is made perfect in weakness."
(2 Corinthians 12:9 NKJV)

For the past three years I have lived out of this verse, learning that God's grace is sufficient regardless of the outcome of Victoria's well-being. Understanding that God's grace extends to the times when I couldn't be the mother that our children needed as I was struggling to keep myself going. This understanding helped reduced the feelings of guilt. Knowing that God's grace is sufficient when you aren't as caring to people around you, especially those closest to you, spouse, extended family and friends, as you used to be, because you are just trying to hold it together to make it through the day.

Don't give up your daily God time

Seek, inquire of and for the Lord, and crave Him and His strength (His might and inflexibility to temptation); seek and require His face and His presence [continually] evermore.
(Psalm 105:4)

As the years have passed the desire in my heart to have more quiet time with God has grown. But there is always the call of everyday tasks, so I have had to be very purposeful about finding that time, actually asking

God where to find that time. He answered me with, 'Get up an hour earlier.'

So 4.30am it was. It is definitely a choice to sit, especially when there was so much around me that was demanding my attention. Sometimes it has been tempting to use that extra waking hour to do the housework. But now if I should miss a day of 'sitting with God' due to a sleep disturbed night, I feel the effects of it all day. I immediately go into operating in Wendy's strength, rather than resting in God's strength.

How to wait

> *Be still and rest in the Lord; wait for Him and patiently lean yourself upon Him (Psalm 37:7 NIV)*

Things happen in God's time, which from my experience seems to be very rarely 'immediately'. Yes it would have been wonderful if Victoria's brain and body had been immediately healed. But that has not been the case. We have to wait. We know Victoria has the victory through what Jesus did for her on The Cross, but we are yet to see the physical manifestation of that healing. Yes it would have been wonderful if the day Victoria finished chemotherapy that everything in our family resumed to normal, but no, that is an individual journey for each of us to reach the place where we can thrive again.

God has gone before us

> *The LORD himself goes before you and will be with you; he will never leave you nor forsake you. Do not be afraid; do not be discouraged.*
> (Deuteronomy 31:8 NIV)

Throughout this journey when we look back, we have been able to see that God has gone before us. The Thank You List that I compiled a few days after Victoria's diagnosis is testament to that. As I have said before I believe it is important to take time to reflect and look for the things to be thankful for, regardless of current circumstances. Finding those things allows us to see how God has indeed gone before us, guiding us, connecting us with people, building skills in us, for purposes that we are completely unaware of. It is another example of His grace in our lives.

Our God is greater

> *How great is our Lord! His power is absolute! His understanding is beyond comprehension!*
> (Psalm 147:5 NLT)

Some amazingly skilled and caring doctors, nurses and therapists have helped Victoria greatly over the past three years. We appreciate all they have done. But I have learned that what the doctor says will happen, isn't always the last word on the situation. There have been aspects of Victoria's journey that we were told what would happen, such as complete hair loss, blood transfusions, Botox, and it has not happened or been required. We are continually learning that God's ways and thoughts are higher than ours (Isaiah 55:8:9) and that He will have the last say. We trust that God's plans for Victoria's future health are different to those of the medical profession.

God will make good come from the bad

> *And we know that God causes everything to work together for the good of those who love God and are called according to his purpose for them.* (Romans 8:28 NLT)

When you are in the middle of a difficult season, particularly if it is a long season, years, it is sometimes very difficult to believe what this verse says. For me, it was one of those scriptures where I had to say many times, 'God, please forgive me for my unbelief and help me to fully believe what this scripture says.'

It was often in complete faith that I declared Romans 8:28, especially in February 2012 when it looked like the residual tumour was growing. At that time I certainly struggled to see any good for our family, each of whom did love God.

But as time has gone on, God has shown me the good

that He is bringing out of this circumstance. We have, through the generosity of charities, had experiences that we wouldn't have had otherwise. As a family, we have developed a compassion for other families with sick children, and some skills in how to help and love those families. We have learnt about patience, and how to love and appreciate each other more. But most importantly, we have grown in our personal relationships with God, relying on Him, more and more. In essence we have matured more into who God has called us to be so we can be better used by Him.

We do not know what awaits Victoria next year, but we know that God's grace is sufficient and that we need to keep seeking Him no matter what. We need to be patient and always remember that He has gone before us. We know that He is greater than any diagnosis and that He will work all things together for good. We will continue to choose to live from the place of victory God has given us through Jesus Christ.

> *But me, I'm not giving up, I'm sticking around to see what God will do. I'm waiting for God to make things right. I'm counting on God to listen to me.* (Micah 7:7 The Message)

If after reading our story, you too would like to live from that place of victory despite your circumstances, then simply say this prayer from your heart, surrendering your life to Jesus Christ. Then seek out a local bible-believing church and connect with other followers of Jesus who can help you on your journey.

> *Lord Jesus, I believe that you are the Son of God. I believe that You became man and died on the cross for my sins. I believe that God raised You from the dead and made you the Saviour of the world. I confess that I am a sinner and I ask you to forgive me, and to cleanse me of all my sins. I accept your forgiveness, and I receive You as my Lord and Saviour. In Jesus' Name I pray. Amen.* [46]

EPILOGUE

It is now almost five years since Victoria stopped chemotherapy treatment in October 2013. So much has happened since then. We have experienced more fear, pain, anger and grief. Yet at the same time we have continued to persevere and overcome in Jesus Name.

God continues to faithfully transform our areas of unbelief into belief, showing us every day that He is trustworthy. He is constantly reminding us of the truth of John 10:10.

> *The thief does not come except to steal, and to kill, and to destroy. I have come that they may have life, and that they may have it more abundantly.* (John 10:10 NKJV)

There are more books in the pipeline, but if you are interested in finding out more about our story, please visit my website wendyrobinson.com.au or contact me at hello@wendyrobinson.com.au

ACKNOWLEDGEMENTS

Writing this story has been a long and sometimes painful journey, re-living many traumatic moments. During this process our ever gracious God has held me in his loving hands, reminding me that it is his story first, and he will bring it to pass in his way and his timing. I am grateful for the gentle guidance of the Holy Spirit, Comforter and Counsellor, who has prompted me with what and when to write, helping me to recall memories that were locked away in pain.

My husband Ken, who has supported me with the time and space to write, knowing that many days dinner would not be cooked and the shirts would not be ironed. I appreciated his marketing expertise in helping this book get to the people who need it the most. Thank you my faithful and clever husband.

Our children, Marshall, Charlotte, Victoria and Alexandra, who have been patient with their Mum's emotional and physical absences. One period that comes to mind is the 2016 Christmas holidays when I spent most mornings locked in our bedroom completing the first draft. Thank you my beautiful children.

My family of origin, who have been a huge support to us throughout this journey, living the pain, grief and victories too. My Mum, my number one supporter, always encouraging me in everything I do; My Dad, often reminding me to make backups of my writing; My sister, who came to my rescue one Saturday afternoon when I was feeling very overwhelmed about creating the photo permissions form. In an hour she reviewed the examples I'd collected and methodically created a form that suited my needs. Thank you for sticking with us.

My Christian brothers and sisters who prayed for me during this project and cheered me on. I am thankful for the words of one friend who after the first year of the project said, 'You know Wendy, it is okay if it takes six years to write this book.' Her words released me to do this project in God's timing, not mine. Most of these friends have not only supported me with this project, but they have lived this journey with us too, some from the beginning when they suggested that something could be very wrong with Victoria. Thank you for your love and grace.

Lake Macquarie Fellowship of Australian Writers, who helped me grow in confidence and competence with my writing. They gently encouraged me during critique meetings as the tears flowed when I re-lived moments of this journey. Thank you for your non-judgemental attitudes as you helped me to tell my story, even though we did not necessarily share the same faith.

Macquarie Life Church Seniors who prayerfully and financially sponsored this project. I am grateful that they chose to use what was in their hands to help get this

ACKNOWLEDGEMENTS

testimony of God's faithfulness out to the wider world. Thank you for believing in me.

Faithful friends who generously gave their time to read and edit this book. I am grateful for all their suggested improvements, knowing that the book is much better because of their input. Thank you for your time and advice.

The graphic designer who God brought back into our lives after seven years. She designed the cover and helped me to get over the final hurdles of designing the book for print and an electronic format. Thank you for helping me push through and complete the project.

This book has not been a one person project. But rather, as with our story itself, it has required a community of people to bring it to pass, all wrapped in the love and perfect timing of our Heavenly Father.

ABOUT WENDY ROBINSON

Wendy Robinson lives in Lake Macquarie, NSW, Australia with her husband Ken and four children. In 2011 their third child, Victoria, then aged three, was diagnosed with a brain tumour. Brain surgery, physical rehabilitation, chemotherapy and emotional trauma became commonplace in their lives.

Wendy drew on her twelve years of project planning in the corporate sphere prior to having children, to develop strategies, processes and checklists to help her family navigate through this season.

Throughout this journey Wendy shared her thoughts and experiences on her blog, which has formed the basis of this book. More than a story, this book is filled with practical survival tactics and tips for parents who find themselves in a similar situation, or people who are struggling with challenging on-going life circumstances.

Born in Auckland, New Zealand, Wendy was blessed with a stable childhood, loved and encouraged by her parents to embrace every opportunity presented to her. A couple of years after completing a Bachelor of Arts degree in Computer Science and Sociology at The University of Auckland she moved to Sydney to further her career. Over the next ten years progressed from working in a computer support role to the manager of Project Management Methodologies at Westpac Banking Corporation. Wendy also completed a Masters of Business and Technology at the University of New South Wales while working full-time.

Wendy accepted Jesus as her Lord and Saviour in 1996 soon after she first met Ken, who ably shared the gospel with her. In 1998, they married, and in 2003 celebrated the birth of their first child, Marshall. Wendy finished work in the corporate sphere to focus on mothering, helping Ken build a sales and marketing business and volunteer at their local church.

In 2005 their second child, Charlotte was born. Under God's direction in 2006 they relocated to Lake Macquarie. Their family continued to grow, with Victoria born in 2007 and Alexandra in 2009. What was to unfold in the coming years left them in no doubt that they were exactly where God wanted them to be.

Today Wendy continues with mothering including supporting her child winning the fight against cancer, working alongside Ken in their business, volunteering at their local church, and still continuing turning to God each day, sometimes each minute, to get the strength required to make it through.

Wendy writes and podcasts a weekly Christian devotion, to find out more, please visit wendyrobinson.com.au

APPENDIX A: SCRIPTURES

He said: "Listen, King Jehoshaphat and all who live in Judah and Jerusalem! This is what the LORD says to you: Do not be afraid or discouraged because of this vast army. For the battle is not yours, but God's. (2 Chronicles 20:15 NIV)

You will not have to fight this battle. Take up your positions; stand firm and see the deliverance the LORD will give you, O Judah and Jerusalem. Do not be afraid; do not be discouraged. Go out to face them tomorrow, and the LORD will be with you. (2 Chronicles 20:17 NIV)

But no weapon that is formed against you shall prosper, and every tongue that shall rise against you in judgement you shall show to be in the wrong. This [peace, righteousness, security, triumph over opposition] is the heritage of the servants of the Lord [those in whom the ideal Servant of the Lord is reproduced]; this is the righteousness of the vindication which they obtain from Me [this is that which I impart to them as their justification], says the Lord. (Isaiah 54:17)

He was wounded for my transgressions, He was bruised for my guilt and iniquities; the chastisement (needful to obtain) peace and well-being for me, was upon Him, and with the stripes (that wounded Him) I am healed and made whole. (Isaiah 53:5)

No test or temptation that comes your way is beyond the course of what others have had to face. All you need to remember is that God will never let you down, He'll never let you be pushed past your limit, He'll always be there to help you through it. (1 Corinthians 10:13 The Message)

Rejoice in the Lord always. I will say it again: Rejoice! Let your gentleness be evident to all. The Lord is near. Do not be anxious about anything, but in everything, by prayer and petition, with thanksgiving, present your requests to God. And the peace of God, which transcends all understanding will guard your hearts and minds in Christ Jesus. (Philippians 4:4-7 NIV)

Cast all your anxiety on him because he cares for you. Be self-controlled and alert. Your enemy the devil prowls around like a roaring lion looking for someone to devour. Resist him, standing firm in the faith, because you know that your brothers throughout the world are undergoing the same kind of sufferings. (1 Peter 5:7-9 NIV)

APPENDIX A: SCRIPTURES

I look up to the mountain – does my help come from here? My help comes from the LORD, Who made the heavens and earth! He will not let you stumble and fall; The one who watches over you will not sleep. Indeed, he who watches over Israel never tires and never sleeps. The LORD himself watches over you! The LORD stands beside you as your protective shade. The sun will not hurt you by day, nor the moon at night, the LORD keeps you from all evil and preserves your life. The Lord keeps watch over you as you come and go, both now and forever. (Psalm 121 NIV)

The thief comes only in order to steal and kill and destroy. I came that they may have and enjoy life, and have it in abundance (to the full, till it overflows). (John 10:10)

For I know the plans I have for you, declares the Lord, plans to prosper you and not to harm you, plans to give you hope and a future. (Jeremiah 29:11 NIV)

Yet amid all these things we are more than conquerors and gain a surpassing victory through Him Who loved us. (Romans 8:37)

But this I recall and therefore have I hope and expectation; it is because of the Lord's mercy and loving kindness that we are not consumed, because His (tender) compassions fail not. They are new every morning; great and abundant is Your stability and faithfulness. The Lord is my portion or share, says my living being (my inner self); therefore I will hope in Him and wait expectantly for Him. (Lamentations 3:21-24)

Faith is the confidence that what we hope for will actually happen; it gives us assurance about things we cannot see. (Hebrews 11:1 NLT)

You are my King and my God who decrees victories for Jacob. Through you we push back our enemies. Through your name we trample our foes. I do not trust in my bow, my sword does not bring me victory; but you give us victory over our enemies, you put our adversaries to shame. In God we make our boast all day long, and we praise your name forever. (Psalm 44:4-8 NIV)

For with God nothing is ever impossible and no word from God shall be without power or impossible fulfilment. (Luke 1:37)

APPENDIX A: SCRIPTURES

Finally, be strong in the Lord and in his mighty power. Put on the full armour of God so that you can take your stand against the devil's schemes. For our struggle is not against flesh and blood, but against the rulers, against the authorities, against the powers of his dark world against the spiritual forces of evil in the heavenly realms. Therefore put on the full armour of God, so that when the day of evil comes, you may be able to stand your ground, and after you have done everything, to stand. Stand firm then, with the belt of truth buckled around your waist, with the breastplate of righteousness in place, and with your feet fitted with the readiness that comes from the gospel of peace. In addition to all this, take up the shield of faith, with which you can extinguish all the flaming arrows of the evil one. Take the helmet of salvation and the sword of the Spirit, which is the word of God. And pray in the Spirit on all occasions with all kinds of prayers and requests. With this in mind, be alert and always keep on praying for all the saints.
(Ephesians 6:10-18 NIV)

APPENDIX B: VICTORIA'S MEDICAL DIAGNOSES

As you read these definitions, please keep in mind all the scriptures of Appendix A, especially Romans 8:37 and Luke 1:37, Our God is greater than these diagnoses.

Brain Cancer

> *Brain cancers include primary brain tumours, which start in the brain and almost never spread to other parts of the body, and secondary tumours (or metastases), which are caused by cancers that began in another part of the body.* [47]

The pathology results indicated that Victoria has a low grade brain tumour, more specifically a pilocytic astrocytoma. For Victoria, the tumour itself is not currently life threatening, praise God. However its location, at the brain stem, makes it very high risk to do a full surgical resection. The brain stem is the non-thinking part of the brain that controls breathing and swallowing.

The American Brain Tumour Association [48] provides this explanation of astrocytomas.

> *Astrocytomas are tumours that arise from astrocytes—star-shaped cells that make up the "glue-like" or supportive tissue of the brain.*
>
> *These tumours are "graded" on a scale from I to*

IV based on how normal or abnormal the cells look. There are low-grade astrocytomas and high-grade astrocytomas. Low-grade astrocytomas are usually localized and grow slowly. High-grade astrocytomas grow at a rapid pace and require a different course of treatment. Most astrocytoma tumours in children are low grade. In adults, the majority are high grade.

Pilocytic Astrocytoma (also called Juvenile Pilocytic Astrocytoma)—These grade I astrocytomas typically stay in the area where they started and do not spread. They are considered the "most benign" (noncancerous) of all the astrocytomas. Two other, less well known grade I astrocytomas are cerebellar astrocytoma and desmoplastic infantile astrocytoma.

Acquired Hemiplegia

The tumour and subsequent stroke during brain surgery has left Victoria with Acquired Hemiplegia.

Hemiplegia [Greek: 'hemi' = half, 'plegia' = loss of function]. Specifically in medical texts, this is defined as 'a one-sided pattern of muscle over-activation and reduction in motor activity, leading to increased muscle tightness, and reflexes, weakness and loss of selective motor control. [49]

APPENDIX B: VICTORIA'S MEDICAL DIAGNOSES

Other clinical problems associated with hemiplegia are epilepsy, sensory, visual, hearing, cognitive, emotional difficulties and secondary physical problems.

Sensory Problems

Victoria's left side is less sensitive to temperature. So we have had to train her to test the bath or shower water with her right hand or foot, to get an accurate gauge of the water temperature.

Visual Field Defect

Victoria has a visual field defect. Initially this was a complete left hemianopia, however over time it appears to be improving.

At least 25% of children with hemiplegia have a visual field defect. This means that their ability to see things in a particular area of vision can be impaired (hemianopia: Greek: 'hemi' = half;' 'anopia' = visual defect). [50]

Secondary Physical problems

Victoria has experienced limited growth in her left arm, hand, leg and foot. They are smaller in length and muscle bulk than her right side.

'With these secondary changes to bone and

muscle two things can happen:

Early on, as the child grows, the affected limbs can grow more slowly. In most children there is a couple of centimetres' difference in true leg length (measure from the top of the bony hip bone – anterior superior iliac spine – to the inside bony bump of the ankle) and perhaps one or two shoe sizes before the age of eight years. It is rare that the difference increases much after that age. The shortening in the arm, hand and fingers can, however, be more pronounced.

Individual muscles and tendons can restrict the amount of movement across joints, a tight contracture can form in them, and the capsule and ligaments of the joint can further restrict movement. However, the risk of the child developing a secondary curvature of the spine is only slightly higher than in the population as a whole.[51]

Additional information

For additional information on hemiplegia, I have found the HemiHelp organisation very helpful. HemiHelp is a charity providing information, support and guidance to people with hemiplegia and their families in the UK. I have purchased some of their resources such as The Hemiplegia Handbook for Parents; Primary Education Pack; Secondary Education Pack. Their website is hemihelp.org.uk

APPENDIX C: OCCUPATIONAL THERAPY ACTIVITIES

These activities are based on our experience. Please get advice from a trained professional occupational therapist before incorporating them into your child's therapy program. Many of these ideas came from the wonderful occupational therapists who have helped Victoria over the years, and we have adapted them to suit our needs.

Therapy Activities

ACTIVITY	Strength	Gross Motor	Fine Motor	Touch Sense
PEG PUZZLE AND SWISS BALL Leaning over the Swiss Ball, supporting body with affected arm and hand (make sure fingers are spread out), do puzzle with normal hand.	✓	✓	✓	
RICE HIDE AND SEEK Hide objects (we sometimes use plastic farm animals) in a container of rice. Child to feel around and find the objects and pull them out.			✓	✓
SHAVING CREAM FINGER PAINTING Spray shaving cream on a plastic tray, and then using affected hand write words, draw pictures, and create shaving cream mountains.			✓	✓
CRAWLING HUNT Cut out 20 of the child's hand prints and put them around the house, with a prize at the end. The child starts at the beginning of the trail, crawling, placing their hands on the handprints, until they reach the prize.	✓	✓		

ACTIVITY	Strength	Gross Motor	Fine Motor	Touch Sense
BALLOON REACHING A helper holds the balloon in various positions, requiring the child to reach for it with the affected arm. Positions include – up high, up high to the left, up high to the right, directly out the front of the child.		✓		
PLAYDOUGH AND MARBLES With the affected hand, push marbles into the playdough, and then pull them out.	✓		✓	

Children's games

To ensure Victoria got the most benefit from these activities we would sometimes put a glove on her right hand, essentially constraining that hand, forcing her to use her left hand.

ACTIVITY	Strength	Gross Motor	Fine Motor	Touch Sense
PEG PUZZLES Using the effective puzzle, pick out and/or place in the pieces of the puzzle.	✓		✓	
TUPPERWARE SHAPE O BALL Pulling the ball apart using two hands. Picking shapes up with affected hands and putting them through the holes in the ball.	✓		✓	
CARD GAMES Shuffling cards, picking up cards, turning cards over, holding cards – all with affected hand.			✓	

APPENDIX C: OCCUPATIONAL THERAPY ACTIVITIES

ACTIVITY	Strength	Gross Motor	Fine Motor	Touch Sense
BOARD GAMES Use the affected hand to shake dice and move tokens. For example Snakes and Ladders, Trouble, Scrabble and Chess.			👌	
PLAYDOUGH AND MODELLING CLAY Pinching with each finger and thumb on affected hand. Rolling, with both hands, to make a snake. Forming the snake into a spiral mat. Rolling balls to make snow men.			👌	🖐
ORIGAMI Using both hands for folds and pressing down on folds.			👌	
KINETIC GAMES Connect 4 – using affected hand to move tokens. Kerplunk – using affected hand to both set up the game and play the game.			👌	
TOY TEA SET Carrying a toy tea set tray with two hands (supination) and gradually increasing the weight on the tray.	🏋	🧍	👌	
BEAN BAGS AND HOOLA HOOPS Throwing bean bags long distance to land in hoop on the ground; or throwing the bean bag up through a hoop. Picking bean bags up with affected hand.	🏋	🧍	👌	
EGG AND SPOON RACES Holding spoon with affected hand (supination).		🧍	👌	
BASKETBALL Can use mini basketball hoop, or full size hoop, focussing on reaching up, throwing and catching.	🏋	🧍		

ACTIVITY	Strength	Gross Motor	Fine Motor	Touch Sense
STICKY BALL GAME Child holds sticky plate with affected hand. Partner throwing the ball in different directions to the child, so the child has to reach in different positions to connect the sticky plate with the ball. Swap and use the affected hand to throw the ball and take the ball off the sticky plate.	✓	✓	✓	✓
BALLOON PUSHES Child turns their affected arm over so their palm faces upwards, and fingers are out-stretched, they push the balloon upwards. If the child is able, count the number of times the balloon is pushed upwards before it falls to the ground.		✓		
BRAIN TEASER PUZZLES Use the affected hand to move and place the puzzle pieces. Examples: IQ Steps – by Smart Games Mini Challenge – 1x3D challenge – by Ionpos Rubicks Cube Addict a ball – especially good for supination and bilateral use			✓	
BEADING Beading can be done to various levels of difficulty, with the goal being the affected hand doing the threading while the normal hand holds the item. Big plastic buttons threaded on wool Smaller buttons threaded on string Jewellery beads threaded on wire			✓	✓

APPENDIX C: OCCUPATIONAL THERAPY ACTIVITIES

ACTIVITY	Strength	Gross Motor	Fine Motor	Touch Sense
STICKERS All types of sticker peeling is helpful, whether it is: - sticker books - peeling off stickers to create pictures and cards - peeling off letter stickers and creating words	✓		✓	
SIMPLE FELT SEWING CRAFTS Pre-packaged felt sewing kits can be purchased at supermarkets and '$2 shops'. These kits are great for developing strength, bi-lateral use and fine motor skills.	✓		✓	✓
BATH CRAYONS Using the affected hand, writing on the bath and tiles, and then using the affected hand to remove the writing.	✓		✓	
LOOM BANDS This craft activity uses small rubber bands to create bracelets and necklaces and more advanced craft items.			✓	
KNUCKLE BONES This old game is particularly good for supination, along with fine motor skills.		✓	✓	

Every day activities

ACTIVITY	Strength	Gross Motor	Fine Motor	Touch Sense
READING A BOOK Holding the book from underneath with two hands (supination) and turning pages with affected hand.			✓	

ACTIVITY	Strength	Gross Motor	Fine Motor	Touch Sense
LIDS Both unscrewing and pulling off lids. Initially may need to loosen the lid.	✓	✓	✓	
COOKING - BAKING COOKIES Holding on to the bowl with affected hand while normal hand does the stirring. Rolling the cookies into balls. Using a fork to press down cookies.	✓	✓	✓	
COOKING - CAKE DECORATING WITH ICING Using the affected hand, squeeze the icing tube to get the icing onto the cake	✓		✓	
COOKING - CUPCAKE DECORATING WITH M&MS Using the affected hand, sort the M&Ms into colour groups and then place the M&Ms on the cupcakes to make patterns. For example, a rainbow; stripes; faces.			✓	
COOKING – PIZZA Starting from making the pizza dough (especially the kneading) right through to putting the toppings on using the affected hand.	✓	✓	✓	✓
COOKING – ROASTING MARSHMELLOWS Use the normal hand to hold the stick Use the affected hand to pick up the marshmellow and put it onto the stick Use the normal hand to cook the marshmellow (or the affected hand if it is strong enough and safe to do so) Use the affected hand to remove the marshmellow from the stick.	✓	✓	✓	✓

APPENDIX C: OCCUPATIONAL THERAPY ACTIVITIES

ACTIVITY	Strength	Gross Motor	Fine Motor	Touch Sense
COOKING – CARRYING TRAYS Carrying a tray with two hands (supination) and gradually increase the weight on the tray.	🏋	🧍	👌	
TECHNOLOGY – TYPING Using the affected hand to type on the keyboard. There are some useful typing programs and apps to assist with this.	🏋		👌	
TECHNOLOGY – IPAD When reading on the iPad, hold the iPad from underneath with two hands (supination) When interacting with iPad use with affected fingers There are also apps available for the specific development of fine motor skills. For example Dexteria.			👌	
EATING - FINGER FOOD Picking up finger food with the affected hand.			👌	✋
EATING – SPECIALISED UTENSILS Using specialised utensils to eat with. For example Victoria has a fork with a moulded handle to help her hand create the right patterns for holding fork.			👌	
SELF-CARE - DRESSING Putting on clothes, doing up buttons and zips.	🏋	🧍	👌	✋
SELF-CARE – SOCKS, SHOES AND LACES Using both hands, putting on socks, shoes and tying shoe laces.	🏋		👌	

ACTIVITY	Strength	Gross Motor	Fine Motor	Touch Sense
SELF-CARE – WASHING HAIR Using both hands for the whole process, from squeezing out the shampoo and conditioner, to using both hands and fingers to massage the head, and then rinsing the shampoo and conditioner out. If it is too hard to do their own hair, encourage them to wash someone else's hair, or even washing a pet.	💪	🕴	👌	🖐
HOUSE WORK - PEGGING OUT WASHING Using affected hand to squeeze pegs both on and off the line. Reaching up to hand out washing.		🕴	👌	
MUSICAL KEYBOARD Using the affected hand to play simple one-handed tunes on the keyboard, making use of all fingers.	💪		👌	
GARDENING – WATERING CAN Holding the watering can in the normal hand, use the affected hand to turn on the tap (or vice versa if necessary) Fill the watering can enough for the affected hand to be able to carry it and water the plants.	💪	🕴		

APPENDIX D: ONE HOUR OCCUPATIONAL THERAPY PLAN

This plan is based on our experience; please get advice from a trained professional occupational therapist before incorporating them into your child's development plan.

ACTIVITY	Timing / Repetitions
SUPINATION STRETCH – FULL EXTENSION Arm fully extended directly in front of the body Palm facing up Ensure shoulders are square and back is straight	Hold the stretch for 30 seconds Repeat three times
SUPINATION STRETCH – BENT AT ELBOW Arm bent at elbow, palm facing up Arm in front of the body Ensure shoulders are square and back is straight	Hold the stretch for 30 seconds Repeat three times
WRIST SUPINATION Arm bent at elbow, palm facing down Wrist flexed up, fingers out straight Ensure shoulders are square and back is straight	Hold the stretch for 30 seconds Repeat three times
BALLOON PUSHING GAME Pump up the balloons with a hand pump Turn the affected hand over with the palm facing up Using the affected hand, push the balloon up to the ceiling Count how many times it is pushed before the balloon touches the ground. Possibly have music playing	5 minutes
EGG AND SPOON GAME Use either a real egg and spoon, or plastic play set Using the affected hand, hold the spoon and egg, walk/run straight ahead. The level of difficulty can be increased by adding obstacles to go around and over	5 minutes

ACTIVITY	Timing / Repetitions
SHOULDER STRENGTHENING – JACK KNIFE ON SWISS BALL Ensure arms are straight up and down Navel pressed in	10 repeats
SHOULDER STRENGTHENING – PUZZLE WILL ON SWISS BALL Roll on the ball Navel pressed in, back straight Affected arm straight and fingers out straight Normal hand doing the puzzle pieces	1, possibly 2 puzzles depending on attention span
SHOULDER STRENGTHENING AND BACK STRETCH Flat back and then round back up (cat stretch) Flat back, opposite arm and leg out, then swap arms and legs	5 repeats
BALLOON REACHING GAME A helper holds the balloon in various positions, requiring the child to reach for it with the affected arm. Balloon positions include – up high, up high to the left, up high to the right, directly out the front of the child.	5 minutes
BASKETBALL DRIBBLING AND CATCHING A helper throwing the ball to different positions requiring the child to reach The child dribbles the ball around cones	5 minutes
FINGER STRENGTHENING AND MOVEMENT Two handed typing on a keyboard. For example on an ipad with an attached keyboard using the Animal typing app.	5 minutes
FINGER STRENGTHENING AND MOVEMENT Story, song or poetry writing using a keyboard, typing with both hands	5 minutes
IN HAND MANIPULATION Using the Connect Four, travel size game, using the normal hand to place a counter in the palm of the affected hand, and then using the affected hand only, manipulate the counter until it is between the thumb and forefinger, then place it in the Connect Four frame	5 minutes

APPENDIX E: MASTER LIST OF LISTS

LIST	PURPOSE
Hospital Emergency Help List	A list of people and phone numbers who have offered to help in times of emergency.
Prayer Warriors	A list of people and mobile phone numbers of people who have offered to pray for us.
On Call Home Support	A list of people and phone numbers of people who are able to come and help at our home if Victoria is in hospital.
On Call Children Sleepovers	For each child, a list of three or four families who are willing to have the child for a sleepover while Victoria is in hospital, to ease the load at home.
Things to do at home before we go to hospital	A list of activities that need to be sorted at home such as preparations for school or work the following day and putting the anaesthetic cream on Victoria's portacath.
Things to do on the way to hospital	A list of activities that need to be sorted at home such as phone calls for cancelling appointments or extra-curricular activities for the next few days.
Things to set up at hospital	A list of items to organise in the hospital room, for example, signs to put on the walls, electronic chargers etc.
On Call Hospital Support – Wendy	A list of people who have offered to visit us in hospital, and possibly sit with Victoria so I can have a break.
On Call Hospital Support – Victoria	A list of Victoria's friends who have offered to visit her in hospital.
Extra-Curricular Activities to cancel	A list of each child's extra-curricular activities and contact numbers
School teachers to notify	Each child's teachers email address to advise what is happening with Victoria and pre-empt any stress that might manifest at school.

LIST	PURPOSE
Victoria's overnight bag packing list	A list of the items Victoria will need for a three day stay in hospital.
Wendy's overnight bag packing list	A list of the items Wendy will need for a three day stay in hospital.
Homecoming checklist	A list of the activities for when Victoria is discharged from hospital.

APPENDIX F: EMERGENCY HOSPITAL BAG CONTENTS CHECKLIST

Victoria's Emergency Hospital Bag Contents

CLOTHES	TOILETRIES
✓ PJ's	✓ Mouthwash
✓ Pull ups & Nappy bags	✓ Toothpaste and toothbrush
✓ Underpants	✓ Shower soap
✓ Clothes	✓ Shampoo and conditioner
✓ Dressing gown	✓ Face cloth
✓ Night boot	
✓ Dirty clothes bag	

FOOD AND DRINK	TOYS, CRAFTS, ELECTRONICS
✓ Drink bottles	✓ Plastic figurines
✓ Rice crackers	✓ Craft activities
✓ Water crackers	✓ Old iPod, charger & headphones
✓ Natural Lollies	

BEDDING	OTHER THINGS
✓ Pillow	✓ Victoria name signs and blu tac
✓ Patchwork blanket	✓ Bible with CDs

Wendy's Emergency Hospital Bag Contents

CLOTHES	TOILETRIES
✓ PJ's	✓ Toothpaste and toothbrush
✓ Bras x3	✓ Shower soap
✓ Underpants x3	✓ Shampoo and conditioner
✓ Clothes x3	✓ Face cloth
✓ Shoes	
✓ Socks and stockings	
✓ Dirty clothes bag	

FOOD AND DRINK	BUSINESS & WRITING EQUIPMENT
✓ Drink bottle	✓ Laptop, mouse, power cable
✓ Microwave container with lid	✓ Business folder
✓ Cutlery	✓ IPAD and earphones
✓ Microwave porridge	✓ Book
✓ Microwave dinners	✓ Bible
✓ Fruit	✓ Journal
✓ Muesli bars	✓ Glasses
	✓ Mobile phone charger

APPENDIX G: HOMECOMING CHECKLIST

Packing up in the hospital room

✓ Take down the Victoria Grace signs
✓ Unmake the parents bed and put dirty linen in the dirty linen room
✓ Remove DVD from the hospital laptop
✓ Unmake Victoria's bed and put dirty linen in the linen room
✓ Text the Prayer Warriors

Things to do in the car

✓ Phone school to notify Marshall and Charlotte that Victoria is out of hospital
✓ Talk with Victoria reminding her that: when we get home Mummy has to spend time with Marshall, Charlotte, Alexandra and Daddy

At Home

✓ Order Takeaway pizza for Homecoming dinner
✓ During dinner thank each family member for how they helped out when Victoria was in hospital
✓ Wash clothes, pillowslip, patchwork blanket, face-cloths and wash bags.
✓ Wash plastic toys
✓ Replenish mouthwash liquids
✓ Replenish shower soap, shampoo and conditioners
✓ Repack Victoria's hospital overnight bag
✓ Repack Wendy's hospital overnight bag

APPENDIX H: SCHOOL BOOKLET

Here is an outline of the contents of a booklet I give to Victoria's teacher each year, along with some examples of the information in the booklet. The content varies from year to year depending on what the current situation is.

School Booklet Content

ITEM	DESCRIPTION
Goals	These goals are defined by Victoria as part of her National Disability Insurance Scheme (NDIS) plan
Appointments	Upcoming appointments with various doctors and therapists, and the next scheduled MRI
Medical Information	Any medical information Chemotherapy regime 38+ Temperature Leg pain Shoulder pain Tiredness AFO (Splint) care
Emotional Health Information and Strategies	Anxiety around scan time Self-esteem and confidence Relief teachers
In the classroom	Eyesight Handwriting Computers
Outside the classroom	Socks, shoes and shoelaces Swimming lessons School Gymnastics Running
Other helpful resources	What about school? Ronald McDonald House Charities Learning Program Guidelines for Teachers – The child with hemiplegia in Primary Education

ITEM	DESCRIPTION
Background information	Our perspective of Victoria Definitions of the brain tumour, acquired hemiplegia

Content Example - Victoria's goals

1. To achieve grade level or higher on school report.

2. To achieve a Gold Medal in the Home Reading program

3. To swing on more than 1 monkey bar

4. To improve my ball skills

5. To not have any pain in my legs

6. To participate in school sporting events

7. To be able to attend school full-time

8. To participate in all school excursions

9. To build up my typing skills so I can type a familiar sentence to the same level as my peers can write it.

APPENDIX H: SCHOOL BOOKLET

Content Example - Medical Information

CHEMOTHERAPY REGIME

Victoria has chemotherapy on Thursdays. Her current schedule is four weeks of treatment and then two weeks break. At this stage, this schedule will continue until July 2013. Chemotherapy is a whole day event at the John Hunter Hospital. Most treatment weeks Victoria is ok on a Friday, just a bit tired. In the first term of 2013, she currently has chemo scheduled for: Thursday 31st January 2013 (Fourth week in the cycle), and then a two week break. She will then commence another four week cycle.

PORTACATH IN LEFT SIDE OF CHEST

Victoria has a portacath inserted under skin on her left upper chest. It looks like a round raised metal button about 2cm in diameter, and has a line going into her heart. The portacath is used for the intravenously administering the chemotherapy. Its presence does not normally bother Victoria. Every four weeks Victoria goes to the hospital for a 'port flush' to ensure the port is working correctly. These appointments are normally after school.

If Victoria falls on her chest, we will need to know as she will have to go to hospital to ensure the portacath has not been damaged.

38 DEGREE + TEMPERATURES

If Victoria has a temperature of 38 degrees or more, she needs to go to the hospital immediately to check for infection. Please call myself or Ken on to make arrangements.

AFO (SPLINT) CARE

Regarding the care of the splint:

- Please don't put it in hot or warm water, or leave it out in the sun – the heat will affect the plastic moulding.

- The splint must be worn with socks

- The splint must not be worn without shoes on.

- The ankle strap on the splint must be tight, the calf strap does not have to be as tight.

- Victoria needs to bend her left leg to put the splint on.

- Sometimes if the splint becomes ill-fitting we use a special plaster (Allevyn thin) to put on Victoria's foot where the splint is rubbing.

APPENDIX H: SCHOOL BOOKLET

Content Example - Emotional Health Information and Strategies

ANXIETY AROUND SCAN TIME

In the three or two weeks prior to the last couple of scans Victoria showed signs of anxiety, mainly presenting as headaches, so whenever possible we try to schedule the MRI's within school holidays. Our current approach to managing this anxiety is:

PRAYING WITH VICTORIA

Scan countdown chart – focussing on all the good things that are happening each day in the two weeks prior to her scan

- Ensuring she is eating and drinking sufficiently

- Distracting her as much as possible with normal activities

- Administering Panadol if the headaches continue

- Arrange the appointment with the oncologist to get the results, to be the day after the scan, rather than having to wait a week.

- We have found that the headaches subside after we have the results of the MRI. If you have any other suggestions re: managing her anxiety please let me know.

SELF-ESTEEM AND CONFIDENCE

Thankfully Victoria has not experienced any bullying at school. However there have been comments made, probably well-meaning, but they do have an impact on Victoria. A common comment by other children is, you can't play this game because you can't run fast. In these situations, we have advised her to go either ignore the comments and join in, or find some other friends to play with.

Victoria sometimes experiences frustration at students asking her about her splint. We have advised her to answer, 'it helps me to walk', however sometimes she has chosen to go with the response, 'I don't want to tell you', which of course is her choice and we respect that.

Victoria is currently involved in various activities to help build self-esteem and confidence. These include swimming with a disabled swimming squad and participating in our church drama & dance group.

RELIEF TEACHERS

Over the last couple of years Victoria struggled when there was a relief teacher in the classroom. The main concern Victoria has is that the relief teacher will not know how to help her if she needs help. Victoria and I have made a half page help note for any relieving teachers with some key information.

Content Example - In the classroom challenges

EYESIGHT

Vision Australia's assessment report of Victoria's vision included the following recommendations for Victoria in the classroom:

- Provide Victoria with a left side, front row seat in all classrooms

- Use black or dark blue marker for whiteboard and overboard projector work to provide the best contrast

- Allow Victoria to leave her seat and move to a close position for board work or viewing and demonstration.

VISUAL FIELD LOSS

Victoria was encouraged to move her eyes and/or head in a systematic manner to scan the immediate environment when trying to locate objects.

- Consider a left margin guide to assist Victoria in locating the next line when reading.

- Victoria may have difficulties seeing people or objects on her left side. Therefore approach Victoria on her right side.

- Provide additional information and time to help Victoria become familiar with new tasks.

HANDWRITING

Due to the acquired hemiplegia (brain injury) Victoria experiences both mental and physical fatigue. (please refer to the Ronald McDonald Learning Program report). Handwriting for any length of time is very tiring both mentally and physically for Victoria. Hence last year she started using an IPAD in class for creative writing activities. The difference in her output was huge. It was if we had found a way to get all the creativity out of her head and onto paper without exhausting her, or her giving up because it was so tiring. The OT has advised that it is important that Victoria still does some handwriting, especially with her spelling words.

When Victoria is doing handwriting she sometimes needs breaks (eg a drink) to rest her hands and then she starts again.

COMPUTERS

Physically she hasn't got the strength and fine motor skills in her left hand to use a normal keyboard for a long period of time. Therefore typing on a normal keyboard is very challenging. So rather than using Typing Tournament, Victoria uses a couple of typing apps on her ipad. The OT was very pleased with the progress Victoria made throughout the year with her typing.

Content Example - Outside classroom challenges

SOCKS AND SHOES AND SHOELACES

Victoria is able to put her socks, splint and shoes on herself, although it is a slow process due to a lack of strength. We encourage her to do this herself as often as possible. However, when she has to have plaster (allevyn thin) on her left foot due to her AFO rubbing, she will need assistance putting on her left sock, so the plaster does not curl up.

Tying shoe laces is challenging for Victoria due to limited strength in her left fingers, she will need assistance with tying her shoelaces.

SWIMMING LESSONS

Victoria has been officially classified as a para-athlete swimmer. She currently trains with a disabled swimming squad. She loves swimming and competes out of school in the state NSW multi-class competitions.

These are some of the impacts Victoria faces

when swimming:

- She cannot straighten her left arm for long periods of time

- She cannot kick equally with both feet for long periods of time

- With the arm length difference, the kickboard work goes a bit askew too, but she does her best.

- She has limited and unbalanced core strength, which makes lying on her back with arms outstretched above her head very difficult.

- She does not currently swim back stroke in her swimming training due to shoulder issues.

It would be preferable if Victoria could use a program prepared by her swimming coach during the school swimming lessons, as it takes the above challenges into consideration. I am happy to come and supervise her if that is required.

SCHOOL GYMNASTICS

Many gymnastic activities are challenging for Victoria as she has reduced movement and strength on her left side (arm, hand, fingers, leg, foot) etc. These impacts include:

APPENDIX H: SCHOOL BOOKLET

- difficulty balancing on her left leg

- difficulty rotating and straightening her left arm.

- reduced strength in left shoulder, arm and hands

Victoria has more stability when she has the splint on, so it is preferable that she wears the splint and shoes during gymnastics. She will need to have close supervision on most of the equipment, especially the balance beam.

Her physio has advised that Victoria should not do any activities involving swinging, until her shoulder is sufficiently strong enough.

RUNNING

Victoria has been officially classified as a para-athlete athlete. Victoria loves running, however her gait is obviously different to most children her age. Regarding Victoria swinging her left leg out when running and walking, her physio has advised,

> 'Her running pattern I think is probably a combination of habit and also weakness. My advice would be to encourage her to not swing her leg out to the side, but to also be aware that she may not be able to correct the position or may only be able to correct the position for a couple of steps. The other thing is that it is going

to be harder for it to correct when she is running to trying to move fast rather than when she is walking.' Physio 9th March 2015.

Our perspective of Victoria

Please remember that despite all these challenges Victoria faces she is a very gusty and determined girl who does not normally think of herself as being sick or disabled.

At home we do not refer to Victoria as being 'sick'. We have endeavoured not to treat Victoria differently from our other three children when it comes to behaviour, obedience and contributing to our family. While we have acknowledged the challenges she faces and the many obstacles she has overcome, (eg at age three Victoria had to re-learn how to make her left hand function) we graciously do not tolerate a 'woe is me' attitude.

Victoria is aware that there is some tumour still in her brain. When we talk about the tumour, we don't refer to the tumour as 'Victoria's tumour'. Rather we tell her that yes, the tumour is there, but it does not belong to her. She knows that Jesus can heal her.

APPENDIX I: SIGNS FOR DISPLAYING AT HOME

These are some of the signs I put around our home to help communicate the importance of reducing the risk of infection to Victoria.

Infection risks and the importance of hand washing

Victoria's Health and Well Being

Anyone outside the immediate family who has these symptoms should be excluded from playing or visiting:

Been exposed to an infection

Has
- an infection
- a runny nose
- a cough
- Diarrhoea
- rash

Hand washing is the single most important way to prevent infection

Symptoms to watch out for

Victoria – Things to watch for

- Thermometer is in the green pen cup
- Temperature is higher than 38 (do not give panadol or neurofen as this may mask a severe infection)
- Do not give Victoria cough mixture
- Exposed to chicken pox, shingles or measles
- Pinpoint red spots, bruising for no reason, bleeding gums, nose bleeds (longer than 10 mins), blood in poos and wees
- Redness around musculums – could be infection
- Redness, swelling, pain or pus at port site. (do not give panadol or neurofen as this may mask a severe infection)

In these instances:
1. On Monday – Thursday after 8.30am ph clinic 4985 5180
2. All other times phone J1 ward 4921 3311 or 4921 3312
3. Put anaesthetic cream (in small black sparkly bag in RedKite bag) on port, cover with gladwrap and seal with micropore tape.
4. Take Victoria & RedKite bag to J1 ward at John Hunter

Doggy Pooping Sign

If you are the owner of the dog that persists in pooing on the grass near our fence, can you please pick up the poo and take it home with you.

Aside from being very inconsiderate leaving the poo behind, you are increasing the risk of infection for our child who receives weekly chemotherapy treatment.

APPENDIX I: SIGNS FOR DISPLAYING AT HOME

Victoria's Mouth Care

> ## Victoria's mouth care
>
> This routine is to be done 4 times a day
>
> 1. Clean teeth with soft toothbrush
> 2. 5mls Sodium Bi-carb mouth wash and SPIT
> 3. 1ml Nilstatyn mouth wash and SWALLOW
> 4. Don't eat or drink for half an hour
>
> If Victoria's mouth becomes sore:
> A. Continue with mouth care program
> B. Drink plenty of water
> C. Can give panadol for the pain
> D. Don't give Neurofen – can cause drop in platelet function
> E. Don't use teething gels – can cause drop in platelet function
> F. If Victoria develops mouth sores, or red or white patches, contact doctor

Victoria's medications

> ## Victoria's Medications
>
> | Day | Medication |
> |---|---|
> | Thursday | Mouthcare – Breakfast, lunch, dinner
Anaesthetic cream 8.30am
Ondansetron liquid – Dinner |
> | Friday | Bactrim x2 – Breakfast, Dinner
Mouthcare - Breakfast, lunch, dinner |
> | Saturday | Mouthcare - Breakfast, lunch, dinner |
> | Sunday | Mouthcare - Breakfast, lunch, dinner |
> | Monday | Bactrim x2 – Breakfast, Dinner
Mouthcare – Breakfast, Afternoon tea, dinner |
> | Tuesday | Mouthcare - Breakfast, Afternoon tea, dinner |
> | Wednesday | Bactrim x2 – Breakfast, Dinner
Mouthcare - Breakfast, Afternoon tea, dinner |

APPENDIX J: HOME MEDICAL KIT

These lists are based on our experience. Please get advice from your oncologist before incorporating them into your home regime.

Equipment

✓ Box with lid for all the chemotherapy related medical equipment
✓ Infra-Red Ear Thermometer
✓ Alcohol wipes
✓ Anti-nausea medication (eg Ondanestron)
✓ Anti-biotics (eg Bactrim)
✓ Mouthcare prevention (eg Nilstatyn, Bi-carbonate soda)
✓ Mouth ulcer treatment (eg Kenalog)
✓ Laxative (eg Lactrolos)
✓ Measuring cups
✓ In the small black sparkly make up bag:
✓ Local anaesthetic cream
✓ Scissors
✓ Tape
✓ Plastic covering
✓ Under the arm digital thermometer

APPENDIX K: CHARITIES THAT HAVE HELPED OUR FAMILY

CHARITY / WEBSITE / DESCRIPTION	PROGRAMS WE HAVE ACCESSED
Camp Quality Australia Campquality.org.au Creating a better life for kids living with cancer	Children's camps Family camps Family fun days Child life therapists Holiday respite house Primary school education program (puppets)
Harry Meyn Foundation Harryshouse.com.au To establish Harry's House in numerous locations to help more families of children living with cancer.	Harry's House at Stockton, Harry's House Mobile Retreat
Kids with cancer Australia Kidswithcancer.org.au A non-profit organisation, a Public Benevolent Institution with over $18.356 million donated to 10 hospitals & thousands of families.	Financial Assistance
Redkite Redkite.org.au Redkite is an Australian cancer charity providing essential support to children and young people (0-24 years) with cancer, and the family and support network who care for them.	Financial assistance Counselling Tele-support groups

CHARITY / WEBSITE / DESCRIPTION	PROGRAMS WE HAVE ACCESSED
Ronald McDonald House Charities Rmhc.org.au An independent non-profit organisation that provides a range of support to seriously ill children and their families when they need it most.	Family room (in hospital) Family Retreats Learning program (tutoring)
Starlight Children's Foundation Australia Starlight.org.au Starlight's mission is "To brighten the lives of seriously ill children and their families".	Starlight Express Room (in hospital) Captain Starlights (in hospital) Wishgranting Family extravaganza days

APPENDIX L: MAINTAINING AND IMPROVING LEG FUNCTION

These lists are based on our experience. Please get advice from your physiotherapist before incorporating them into your home regime.

Activities and definition

ACTIVITY	DEFINITION / EXPLANATION
Physiotherapy	The treatment of disease, injury, deformity, etc., by physical methods including manipulation, massage, infrared heat, remedial exercise, etc., not by drugs. (The Australian Concise Oxford Dictionary, third edition)
Hydrotherapy	The use of water in the treatment of disorders, usually exercises in swimming pools for arthritic or partially paralysed patients. (The Australian Concise Oxford Dictionary, third edition)
Hippotherapy	A movement therapy with the help of the horse (Greek 'Hippos' = horse)
Horse Riding	Weekly riding program at a local Riding for the Disabled centre
Stretching	We use a range of activities to help with stretching. • Sustained 20 minute stretches of left calf and hamstring muscles. • Stretching on the wedge board • Over-night stretching in the night boots • Serial casting
Swimming	Swimming training in a specialised squad for disabled swimmers.

Equipment

Over the years we have purchased a few things to help Victoria with her legs and feet.

ACTIVITY	DEFINITION / EXPLANATION
Ankle Foot Orthosis	A brace usually made of plastic, that is worn on the lower leg and foot to support the ankle, hold the foot and ankle in the correct position and correct foot drop. Abbreviated AFO. Also known as foot drop brace. (medicinenet.com)
Calf Stretching Wedge	A wooden box with 45 degree slopping lid
BOSU Balance Trainer	The BOSU Balance Trainer is, quite simply, a piece of exercise equipment that resembles a ball, cut down the middle. It's made of a rubber bladder on a stiff non-slip and non-marking base. The bladder is inflated until the bladder resembles half a ball. (Optomo.com.au)
Allevyn thin	Allevyn* Thin is a self-adhesive, water resistant dressing that promotes a moist wound environment and can be left on a wound for up to 5 days. (smith-nephew.com) We have found this to be a wonderful plaster when Victoria has experienced rubbing or blisters on her foot.
Organic Cold/ heat packs	We use the Heat Bags plus brand – 100% Western Australian Lupin, not treated with chemicals, fully handwashable, forms to your body shape, 99% allergy free, gluten free. We have three of these at home, one at school and one at kid's church.

APPENDIX L: MAINTAINING AND IMPROVING LEG FUNCTION

ACTIVITY	DEFINITION / EXPLANATION
My Moves Exercises for children with hemiplegia DVD	This DVD is produced by HemiHelp. 'My Moves is a fun exercise aid for kids with hemiplegia and their parents. Suitable for children aged 0-13+, this DVD is packed full of exercises that encourage use of both sides, build muscle strength, improve posture and encourage a wide range of movement.' (Hemihelp)

NOTES

[1] Rainey D & Rainey B, 2007, Moments with You, Daily connections for couples, Regal Books, Ventura, CA, USA, 7

[2] Omartian S 1997, The Power of a Praying Wife, Harvest House Publishers, Eugene, OR, USA, 24-25.

[3] Sherrer Q & Garlock R 1992, The Spiritual Warrior's Prayer Guide – using God's Word in prayer and spiritual warfare, Vine Books, USA, 18.

[4] Meyer, J 1995, Battlefield of the Mind: Winning the Battle in Your Mind, Harrison House, Inc. Tulsa, OK, USA, 56.

[5] Cartledge, David 1997, The person and work of the Holy Spirit, Paraclete Productions, Australia, 3.

[6] Swindoll, Charles R 1993, Flying closer to the flame - A Passion for the Holy Spirit, Word Incorporated, Dallas, TX, USA, 13.

[7] Meyer, J 1995, Battlefield of the Mind: Winning the Battle in Your Mind, Harrison House, Inc. Tulsa, OK, USA, 42.

[8] Barnes, L and Fairhurst C 2011, The Hemiplegia Handbook for parents and professionals, Mac Keith Press, London, UK, 40.

[9] Westberg, G 1992, Good Grief: A Constructive Approach to the Problem, Joint Board of Christian Education, Australia

[10] Barnes, L and Fairhurst C 2011, The Hemiplegia Handbook for parents and professionals, Mac Keith Press, London, UK, 39.

[11] Ibid, 39.

[12] Camp Quality, https://www.campquality.org.au (accessed 5th February 2016)

[13] Franklin, J 2008, Fasting, Charisma House, FL, USA, 9-11.

[14] Ibid, 14

[15] Voskamp, A 2010, One Thousand Gifts: a dare to live fully right where you are, Zondervan, Grand Rapids, MI, USA, 21.

[16] Marshall, C 1974, Something More, In search of a deeper faith, Chosen Books Publishing Company, Lincoln, VA, USA

[17] Voskamp, A 2010, One Thousand Gifts: a dare to live fully right where you are, Zondervan, Grand Rapids, MI, USA

[18] Kidsmatter Early Childhood Team, 'Supporting Parents

NOTES

and Carers to look after themselves,' https://www.kidsmatter.edu.au/sites/default/files/public/KMECC3-201208-Supporting-to-%20look-after-themselves.pdf (accessed 6th May 2016)

[19] I and M Grant, Growing Great Girls: How to bring out the best in your daughter, 2008, Random House New Zealand, 35.

[20] Steiner Rice, H 1970, Lovingly Poems for all seasons, Baker Book House Company, Grand Rapids, MI, USA, 53.

[21] Redkite, Information for parents and family members, Redkite, Australia

[22] Steiner Rice, H 1970, Lovingly Poems for all seasons, Baker Book House Company, Grand Rapids, MI, USA, 57.

[23] Baikie, K and Wilhelm K, 'Emotional and physical health benefits of expressive writing,' Advances in Psychiatric Treatment 2005, 11 (5) 338-346 http://apt.rcpsych.org/content/11/5/338 (accessed 2nd January 2017)

[24] Cancer.net, Astrocytoma – Childhood Guide, http://www.cancer.net/cancer-types/astrocytoma-childhood (accessed 13th February 2013)

[25] Busch, W, http://izquotes.com/quote/28347 (accessed 9th January 2017)

[26] Boyer, K, 'Silent Strong Dad,' https://www.bustle.com/articles/90675-5-fathers-day-poems-that-will-inspire-you-to-tell-your-dad-just-how-much-you (accessed 9th January 2017)

[27] Westberg, G 1992, Good Grief: A Constructive Approach to the Problem, Joint Board of Christian Education, Australia

[28] Burpo T, Burpo S, 2011, Heaven is for Real for kids, Tommy Nelson, Colorado Springs, CO, USA

[29] Redkite, Information for parents and family members, Redkite, Australia, 5.

[30] Redkite, Information for parents and family members, Redkite, Australia, 3.

[31] Stone, N 1944, Names of God, Moody Publishers, Chicago, IL, USA, 58.

[32] C Tomlin, How great is our God, 2011

[33] Nolte, D L, 'Children learn what they live,' Http://www.blinn.edu/socialscience/LDThomas/Feldman/Handouts/0801hand.htm (accessed on 16th May 2013)

[34] Stone, N 1944, Names of God, Moody Publishers, Chicago, IL, USA, 81.

NOTES

[35] Marshall, C 1974, Something More, In search of a deeper faith, Chosen Books Publishing Company, Lincoln, VA, USA

[36] Red Cross Australia, https://www.donateblood.com.au/red25 (accessed on 28th March 2017)

[37] Osteen, J 2012, I declare, 31 promises to speak over your life, FaithWords, New York, NY, USA, vii.

[38] J Meyer, The Everyday Life Bible, 2006, FaithWords, Hachette Book Group, New York, NY, USA, 1483.

[39] McCoy, M, 'Top 10 Benefits of Charitable Giving and Donations,' www.moneycrashers.com (accessed on 8th January 2017)

[40] L Hodges & S Buchanan, Angels watching over me, 2005, Zonderkids, Grand Rapids, MI, USA

[41] Redkite, Information for parents and family members, Redkite Australia

[42] I Grant, Growing Great Boys – 100s of practical strategies for bringing out the best in your son, 2006, Random House New Zealand, 193.

[43] Ibid, 197.

[44] Prince, D 2010, God's Word Heals, Derek Prince

Ministries, International, USA.

[45] I Grant, Growing Great Boys – 100s of practical strategies for bringing out the best in your son, 2006, Random House New Zealand

[46] Gerald, K 1997, The Proving Ground - Nine tests that prove your personal potential, Insight Publishing Group, Tulsa, OK, 106.

[47] Cancer Council Australia, 'Brain Cancer,' http://www.cancer.org.au/about-cancer/types-of-cancer/brain-cancer.html (accessed 12th January 2017)

[48] American Brain Tumour Organisation, 'Astrocytoma' (http://www.abta.org/brain-tumor-information/types-of-tumors/astrocytoma.html) (accessed 12th January 2017)

[49] Barnes, L and Fairhurst C 2011, The Hemiplegia Handbook for parents and professionals, Mac Keith Press, London, UK, 17.

[50] Ibid, 32.

[51] Ibid, 35.

www.ingramcontent.com/pod-product-compliance
Lightning Source LLC
Chambersburg PA
CBHW032022290426
44110CB00012B/627